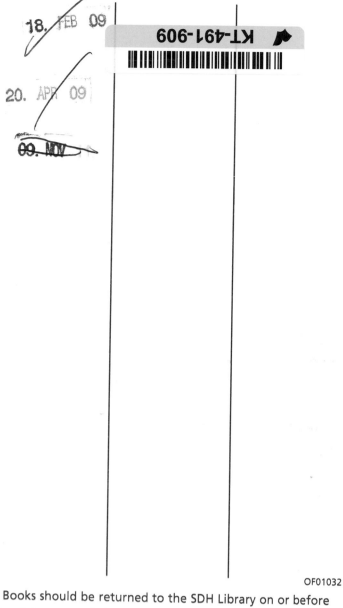

Emergency Vascular Surgery
A Practical Guide

Eric Wahlberg   Pär Olofsson   Jerry Goldstone

Emergency Vascular Surgery

A Practical Guide

With 68 Figures and 39 Tables

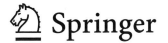 Springer

Eric Wahlberg, MD, PhD
Associate Professor
Karolinska Institute and University Hospital
Department of Vascular Surgery
17176 Stockholm
Sweden

Pär Olofsson, MD, PhD
Associate Professor
Karolinska Institute and University Hospital
Department of Vascular Surgery
17176 Stockholm
Sweden

Professor **Jerry Goldstone, MD**
University Hospital of Cleveland
Case Western Reserve
Division of Vascular Surgery
Cleveland, Ohio 44106
USA

ISBN   978-3-540-44393-3 Springer Berlin Heidelberg New York

Library of Congress Control Number: 2006936731

Springer is a part of Springer Science + Business Media
springer.com

© Springer-Verlag Berlin Heidelberg 2007

Editor: Gabriele M. Schröder, Heidelberg, Germany
Desk Editor: Stephanie Benko, Heidelberg, Germany
Production: LE-TeX Jelonek, Schmidt & Vöckler GbR, Leipzig, Germany
Drawings: Medical Art, Gudrun and Adrian Cornford, Reinheim, Germany
Typesetting: am-productions GmbH, Wiesloch, Germany
Cover design: Frido Steinen-Broo, eStudio Calamar, Spain

Printed on acid-free paper   24/3180 YL – 5 4 3 2 1 0

Preface

Emergency Vascular Surgery – A Practical Guide provides a concise guide to managing patients with all kinds of emergent vascular problems. It is not intended to be a "classic" textbook, so the background information given is very concise. The focus is instead on management and treatment, especially open surgical strategies.

The text is written for newcomers to the vascular surgical field, for surgical trainees, and for all doctors who treat emergent vascular surgical patients in the emergency department. We believe the hands-on approach and the practical tips will be appreciated by these readers in the clinical situation, and we hope the book may also serve as a quick review before a physician takes care of a case. Medical students during surgical clerkships might find parts of the book valuable, as will experienced vascular surgeons.

The book is organized into two sections: specific body areas and general concepts. The former covers the body from head to toe and includes separate chapters for injuries and for nontraumatic disease. In the second part, some general principles related to emergency vascular surgical practice are discussed. Management of complications is difficult to cover in a book of this scope, so the principles given in the chapter pertaining to this area are not very detailed. The final chapter gives general vascular surgical guidelines for the inexperienced surgeon.

All chapters are organized the same way. They start with a brief background that aims to motivate the reader and give an idea of incidence and pathophysiology. The rest of the chapter follows the patient's course through the hospital: The clinical presentation is followed by suggestions for work-up and diagnosis, and the next part concerns management and treatment – emergency treatment, selection of patients for emergency surgery, and ways to perform common vascular surgical procedures. Technical tips on complicated procedures are also provided. Finally, the chapters end with a brief summary on management after treatment, with some examples of outcome and results. Most chapters also contain illustrations to facilitate the technical description of the surgical procedures and notes to highlight particularly important aspects. A few references for further reading are also suggested; they have been selected to give a better understanding of the issues and do not necessarily refer to information given in the text.

The authors would like to acknowledge and thank a number of people involved in the writing of this book. First, we are grateful to the initial authors of the Swedish book from 1998 that gave us the idea to expand its contents and write an English version of it. Thank you all for letting us continue in this direction. We are also very grateful to all the residents, vascular trainees, and vascular surgeons who have read chapters and given us valuable suggestions on how to improve the content and structure. Last but not least, we acknowledge the secretaries Annika Johansson and Synnove Nordstrom for all of their help with this project.

Eric Wahlberg
Pär Olofsson
Jerry Goldstone
Stockholm and Cleveland 2007

Contents

Specific Areas

PART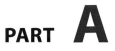

Vascular Injuries to the Neck

1

CONTENTS

1.1 Summary

- Severe vascular injury after blunt neck trauma can be present even in the absence of clinical signs.
- Be liberal with duplex or angiography after blunt trauma when cervical vessel injuries cannot be ruled out.
- Associated injuries on the cervical spine, airway, and digestive tract must always be considered.
- Always stabilize the neck of patients in all types of severe cervical trauma until the entire spectrum of injuries is known.
- If the patient is stable angiography should always be performed in penetrating injuries to zones I and III.
- If available, duplex or angiography is recommended in zone II injuries in order to select between conservative and surgical management.

1.2 Background

Traumatic injuries to the cervical vessels are relatively uncommon and constitute only about 5–10% of all vascular injuries. In about 25% of patients with blunt head and neck trauma, the cervical vessels are involved. The most common mechanism is penetrating injuries, but the incidence of blunt vascular trauma is probably underestimated because related symptoms are often vague and not recognized. The patients are mostly young, and despite the low incidence, mortality and morbidity are very high. Mortality is, in most series, between 5% and 40%, and persistent neurological consequences are reported in up to 80% of patients. Mortality is not only caused by massive bleeding and cerebral ischemia due to embolization or thrombotic occlusion associated with the vascular injury, but also secondary damage to the aerodigestive tract (e.g., airway compression from a large expanding hematoma).

The anatomical location and the often complex associated injuries make traumatic cervical vascular injuries extremely challenging.

1.2.1 Causes and Mechanism

1.2.1.1 Penetrating Trauma

The most common mechanism for cervical vascular injuries is penetrating trauma. As shown in Table 1.1, the common carotid is the most frequently injured major artery. The type of penetrating trauma is most often stab wounds by knives, but other mechanisms are high- or low-velocity projectile and gunshot wounds, and bone fragments from fractures. High-velocity penetrating trauma can also cause secondary "blunt" injuries by a shock wave.

1.2.1.2 Blunt Trauma

Blunt trauma to the cervical vessels is thought to be less than 0.5% of all blunt traumas to the body, but recent reports indicate that many blunt vascular injuries go undetected.

Table 1.1. Frequency of vessel and associated organ injuries in penetrating injuries to the neck

Site of injury		
Major vessels		
Arteries	Common carotid artery	73%
(10–15%)	Internal carotid artery	22%
	External carotid artery	5%
Veins	External jugular	50%
(15–25%)	Internal jugular	50%
Other organs		
Digestive tract	5–15%	
Airway	4–12%	
Major nerves	3–8%	
No involvement of important structures	40%	

The internal carotid artery is involved in more than 90% of these injuries, most commonly its distal parts. Three to ten percent of all carotid injuries are caused by blunt trauma. The true incidence is unknown, but a few reports cite figures in the range of 0.1–1.1% of all blunt head and neck injuries. The variation is related to the type of study performed and methodology used; some studies are retrospective, while others use screening with angiography or computed tomography (CT). Blunt carotid injuries occur in motor vehicle, industrial accidents or after assaults. Injuries to the vertebral artery are less common because they are well protected by osseous structures. Injuries to the vertebral arteries are most commonly caused by intraoral trauma dislocated fractures or penetrating trauma. The mechanisms are the same as in the internal carotid artery.

The mechanism of injury is either a direct blow or hyperextension and rotation of the neck. In the latter type, the internal carotid artery is stretched over the body of the C2 vertebra and the transverse process of C3, which causes an intimal flap with subsequent risk for embolism or dissection and thrombotic occlusion. Other consequences are development of a pseudoaneurysm or, in rare cases, even complete disruption of the internal carotid at the base of the skull. In some reports, up to 50% of patients are reported to have bilateral vascular injuries after blunt trauma to the neck. Carotid dissection is also reported to occur after minor head and neck trauma, and to be associated with activities such as unaccustomed physical exercise; "heading" a soccer ball and childbirth.

1.3 Clinical Presentation

Common to all neck trauma is that many patients with severe vascular or other injuries present with a clinical picture deceptively lacking obvious symptoms and signs of their injuries. Furthermore, significant associated intracranial lesions, multiple organ injuries, and alcohol or drug intoxication often confuse the clinical picture. The history and clinical examination must be performed with a high level of suspicion in order to achieve a good platform for the diagnostic evaluation and management.

1.3.1 Medical History

Knowing the mechanism of injury can provide important clues to the type of and potential vascular injury. Information about the type and extent of trauma should be obtained from the patient, paramedics, or relatives. In penetrating injuries, information about external bleeding is important: the magnitude and volume (brisk and pulsating or oozing), the color (dark venous or bright arterial), and the duration (initial but stopped or ongoing). In cases of brisk bleeding, injuries to the carotid artery or larger veins are likely. Symptoms of hypovolemia or shock during the course from incident to admission indicate significant blood loss. Respiratory problems indicates the presence of a large hematoma compressing the airway, which could require immediate attention and management. A history of a symptom-free interval of hours or days from the injury to the appearance of neurological symptoms is common after blunt carotid trauma. A frequent type of symptom is a typical transient ischemic attack but complete stroke or amaurosis fugax also occurs.

Because the carotid is the most common injured artery, it is essential to assess the patient's mental status, including possible alterations during transport as well as transient, progressive, or permanent focal neurological changes. It is also important to inquire about symptoms related to associated cranial nerve injuries (see Table 1.2).

Difficulties or pain with swallowing suggest an esophageal injury and should increase the suspicion for associated vascular injuries. In blunt carotid injuries, headache and/or cervical pain are the most common symptoms, followed by symptoms indicating cerebral or retinal ischemia (see Table 1.3). Neck wounds or bleeding from the

Table 1.2. Examples of findings and symptoms in neck injuries

Injury type		Signs	Symptoms
Vascular penetration			
Artery or vein		Bleeding, hematoma, swelling	Bleeding, pain
Carotid or vertebral		Horner's syndrome[a]	Hanging eye lid, headache
Bleeding with tracheal compression		Stridor, supraclavicular and intercostal retractions	Dyspnea
Embolization		Hemiplegia/hemiparesis	Weakness, numbness
Arteriovenous fistula		Bruit or thrill	Swelling
Cranial nerves			
Glossopharyngeal nerve	IX	Pharyngeal paresis, soft palate hanging down	Difficulty swallowing
Vagal nerve	X	Vocal cord paresis	Hoarseness
Accessory nerve	XI	Unable to shrug the shoulders	Weakness
Hypoglossal nerve	XII	Tongue deviation toward the injured side	Difficulty swallowing
Aerodigestive tract			
		Subcutaneous emphysema	Shortness of breath. Difficulty or pain with swallowing
		Hemoptysis	
Mandibular fracture		Tenderness	Pain, difficulty speaking

[a] Caused by disruption of the blood supply (vasa vasorum) to the superior cervical ganglion or by direct injury to the sympathetic nerve plexus

Table 1.3. Consequences of blunt injuries to the carotid artery

Type of injury	Mechanism	Consequences	Symptoms/signs
Direct blow	Rupture	Hematoma	Swelling and respiratory problems
		Pseudoaneurysms	Bruit, swelling
	Intimal tear	Thrombosis	Stroke, focal neurology
Rotation-extension	Intimal tear	Dissection	Stroke, focal neurology
		Thrombosis	Stroke, focal neurology

mouth, nose, or ears after severe blunt cervical trauma may be associated with injuries to the vertebral artery.

1.3.2 Clinical Signs

A penetrating injury is usually obvious at inspection of an open wound with signs of recent or ongoing bleeding. A "sucking wound" suggesting a connection with the aerodigestive tract indicates an increased risk for "proximity" injuries to the major cervical arteries (i.e., the vertebral arteries). Even minor external signs of penetrating trauma can be associated with a severe underlying vascular injury. One example is the expanding hematoma. The reverse however, is also possible – a large hematoma compressing adjacent structures harbored by the stiff fascial layers of the neck but undetectable at inspection. Sometimes signs of airway obstruction reveal such injuries. Signs and symptoms of penetrating cervical vascular trauma are summarized in Table 1.2.

Half of the patients with significant blunt vascular injuries to the neck lack symptoms at admission but develop symptoms and signs within 24 h. In blunt trauma, it is therefore important to perform a careful neurological examination at admission to obtain a baseline for later comparisons at the mandatory repeated examinations. The neurological evaluation should seek signs of central as well as peripheral nerve injuries – alertness, motor and sensory function, reflexes in the extremities – as well as signs of cranial nerve dysfunction (Table 1.2). It is important to thoroughly inspect for signs of contusion, asymmetry, or deformity that indicate underlying hematomas and to note the hematoma size for later estimation of possible expansion. Other physical findings indicating a

vascular injury are tenderness over the carotid artery and in the scalp. The most common associated injury is fracture of the mandible.

NOTE
The physical examination can be negative despite severe vascular injury after blunt cervical trauma.

1.4 Diagnostics

1.4.1 Penetrating Trauma

The location of penetrating cervical injuries are generally divided into three different zones that are helpful for planning the diagnostic work-up and management (Fig. 1.1). It is therefore important to classify the localization of the injury into zones according to this subdivision. The rationale for this lies in difficulties achieving proximal control in zone I injuries and distal control in zone III. Exploration and the possibility of obtaining control are much easier in zone II injuries.

Patients with "hard signs" of major vessel injury – shock, active brisk bleeding, rapidly expanding hematoma (for discussion about the definition of "expanding hematoma," see Chapter 12, p. 149) – and those with neurological deficit or severe airway obstruction should be transported to the operating room for immediate exploration and treatment.

Patients with "soft signs" of major vessel injury – history of bleeding, stable hematoma, and/or cranial nerve injury – usually need further work-up. This is also true for patients who don't have signs, but who have an injury in proximity to major vessels. This group constitutes the majority of penetrating neck injuries. The following recom-

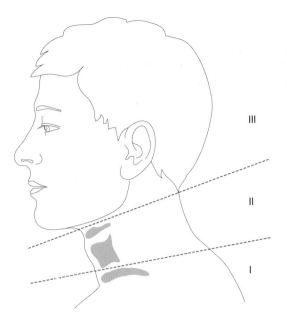

Fig. 1.1. Division of the neck into three zones aids in the management of penetrating cervical vascular injuries (Monson DO, Saletta JD, Freeark RJ. Carotid-vertebral trauma. J Trauma 1969; 9:987–999). Zone I extends inferiorly from 1 cm above the manubrium to include the thoracic outlet; zone II extends from the upper limit of zone I to the angle of the mandible; and zone III is between the angle of the mandible and the base of the skull

mendations have been generally accepted in these cases:

Zones I and III: With the exception of unstable patients, angiography is always indicated. The goals are detecting injury, planning an operation possibly requiring special exposures (e.g., intrathoracic clamping), and excluding indications for operation.

Zone II: Injuries penetrating the platysma in this zone require surgical exploration to identify and treat vascular injuries as well as injuries to the aerodigestive tract unless the patient is asymptomatic and angiography, duplex ultrasound, and CT have ruled out such injuries.

Duplex ultrasound in the hands of an experienced examiner has been shown to be consistent with angiography findings in more than 90% of cases. It can reveal dissections, thrombotic occlusion, intimal flaps, pseudoaneurysms, and hema-

tomas. Altered flow patterns indicating high resistance or abnormal turbulence can be associated with a lesion distally in the internal carotid artery. The developing experience of the duplex technique has prompted a policy change in some hospitals, and duplex ultrasound is used as the primary diagnostic tool for all injuries in stable patients. This examination is performed prior to the decision about angiography or surgical exploration and irrespective of anatomic zone. In some centers, therapeutic decisions are based on thin-slice high-speed CT scans instead.

Gunshot wounds deserve special comment. All patients with such injuries should be screened with angiography or duplex ultrasound. Because associated injuries are common, CT scanning of the head, surgical spine, and aerodigestive tract should also be included in the diagnostic work-up.

NOTE
Injuries not penetrating the platysma need no further vascular evaluation.

1.4.2 Blunt Trauma

The diagnosis of vascular injuries after blunt trauma is much more challenging. As previously noted, clinical signs and symptoms are frequently subtle or absent, and initial transient or late neurological deficits are common. The most commonly injured vascular segment is the distal internal carotid artery. Dissection, with varying degrees of luminal narrowing, is the most common injury. Other types are pseudoaneurysm or even total transection of the artery with free extravasation. If an expert ultrasonographer is available, duplex ultrasound can be considered as a primary screening method, but a negative study cannot be relied upon to exclude the presence of a clinically significant injury. For all other patients, the recommendation is angiography as the first option, as it is still the gold standard.

In all patients with basilar skull fractures, unstable cervical spine fractures, Horner's syndrome, or LeFort-II or-III facial fractures, recent studies advocate a more aggressive attitude with angiographic screening for blunt carotid injuries. Extracranial carotid injuries are also reported to be

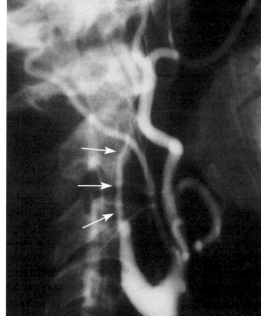

Fig. 1.2. Angiography showing a dissection of the internal carotid artery resulting in a narrowing of the lumen with the typical "string sign" appearance (*arrows*)

more common in patients with a Glasgow coma scale of 8 or less and thoracic injury. A typical finding at angiography in caroid dissection is a stenosis, irregular and often tapered, beginning 2 or 3-cm distal to the bifurcation and often extending up to the base of the skull, above which it is abruptly reconstituted with a normal lumen. Occasionally a typical "string sign" can be seen in the stenosed segment (Fig. 1.2).

CT is not reliable for diagnosing blunt cervical vascular injuries. CT angiography is under development and is likely to play a greater role in the future. It has the advantage of short examination times and concurrent diagnosis of other injuries, such as brain injuries and skull or facial fractures. Magnetic resonance imaging (MRI) has a high sensitivity and specificity in relation to angiography (95% and 99%, respectively) for detecting blunt carotid injuries, as does MR angiography (84% and 99%), but both are time-consuming and complicate monitoring and resuscitation of the critically injured patient.

NOTE
> A patient with neck trauma and a possible vascular injury who is stable, has stabilized after resuscitation, or has a transcervical gunshot injury should undergo a selective aortic arch angiography.

1.5 Management and Treatment

1.5.1 Management Before Treatment

1.5.1.1 Management in the Emergency Department

As with other major trauma, the Advanced Trauma Life Support guidelines should be followed for severe cervical vascular injuries. Consequently, airway and respiration have first priority, followed by control of bleeding. Control of bleeding is best achieved by external finger or manual compression applied directly to the bleeding site. Blindly applied clamps should not be attempted because of the risk of iatrogenic injuries to blood vessels as well as to other organs.

Resuscitation to hemodynamic stability is important. Hypertension may increase bleeding and also induce progress of a dissection, while hypotension will increase the risk for thrombosis and cerebral malperfusion.

1.5.1.2 Airway Obstruction

Patients with neck trauma and airway obstruction require meticulous management and close cooperation with the anesthesiologist. Intubation should be performed in an anesthetized patient to avoid gagging, which might discharge clots and thus cause profuse bleeding or embolization. Caution should also be taken when the patient's neck is flexed at the intubation because of the risk of associated cervical vertebral fractures. There is an obvious risk for dislocation and spinal injury. The intubation might also be technically challenging because a large hematoma might cause total compression of the trachea. Emergency tracheotomy or coniotomy is then the only alternative, but it may also be complicated by the deranged anatomy and risk of bleeding. The risk of profuse uncontrolled bleeding is greatest if the hematoma is located on the anterior aspect of the neck because the tamponade will be immediately lost when the pretracheal fascia is incised. By using liberal intubation early on and under controlled conditions, such situations could be avoided.

1.5.1.3 Immediate Operation or Further Diagnostic Work-up?

The surgeon has to decide in the emergency department whether the patient requires immediate operation, further diagnostic examination, or continued observation.

It is important to emphasize that although standard teaching has been that exploration is required for all zone-II injuries that penetrate the platysma, as well as for gunshot wounds that cross the midline, the availability of better diagnostic modalities has permitted the use of selective exploration protocols.

The following recommendations are given for this initial selection:

1. Immediate operation is indicated for unstable patients with active bleeding not responsive to vigorous resuscitation or with rapidly expanding hematoma or airway obstruction, irrespective of anatomical zone.
2. Injuries in zone II not penetrating the platysma need no further examination.
3. All others require further diagnostic evaluation with angiography, duplex ultrasound, and CT to determine whether critical structures have been injured. If angiography or high-quality duplex ultrasound is not available, injuries in zone II need to be surgically explored.

Depending on the results of these diagnostic studies, the following general recommendations can be given regarding management of vascular injuries.

Repair is recommended in all patients with penetrating carotid injuries when there is still evidence of prograde flow and the patient has no major neurological symptoms. For minor injuries to the carotid artery, including those with small but adherent intimal flaps, defects, or pseudoaneurysms <5 mm in size, repair is recommended in symptomatic patients. If the patient is asymptomatic and there is no ongoing active bleeding, a conservative approach has proven to be a safe alternative. The patient needs to be followed on an inpatient basis for a couple of days to monitor for the appearance of neurological symptoms. Liberal indications for repeated duplex examination are

employed. Anticoagulation therapy, antiplatelet therapy, or both should also be initiated.

Management of significant carotid artery injury existing with major neurological deficit and coma is controversial. Some surgeons suggest only observation and palliation, especially in patients with CT-verified cerebral infarction, because of the poor prognosis. Others advocate repair. This standpoint is based on the difficulties of deciding whether the vascular trauma, cerebral contusion, or drugs caused the coma. Some reports, however, indicate a possibility of better outcome after exploration and repair.

When the carotid artery is occluded and there are no neurological symptoms, observation and anticoagulation with heparin followed by 3 to 6-months of coumadin is a general treatment irrespective of the type of trauma. In patients with major neurological symptoms and a verified infarction on CT, anticoagulation is associated with a considerable risk for bleeding. The patients prognosis is then poor, and palliation is recommended.

In blunt trauma, indications for exploration and open repair are rarer due to the mostly distal location of injuries to the internal carotid artery. For asymptomatic injuries, including dissection, anticoagulation is usually the only treatment needed and is indicated to prevent thrombosis of the injured segment and/or embolization from it. Only injuries that after angiography appear to be easily accessible during surgery and are symptomatic should be considered for repair. This is particularly important when there appears to be a high risk for embolization. In patients with decreased consciousness having an occluded internal carotid artery after blunt trauma and with no, or with severe, neurological symptoms, most reports advocate only observation without surgical exploration. As already mentioned, however, some do recommend a more aggressive approach. This strategy requires extensive experience in carotid surgery.

1.5.1.4 Which Patients Can Be Safely Transported?

Because cervical vascular injuries often require an experienced vascular surgeon, a thoracic surgeon, an endovascular specialist, and frequently also a specialist in head and neck surgery, some patients would benefit from being transported to a hospital where such expertise is available. A stable patient can be transported to another hospital after intubation, or with readiness for emergency intubation in the ambulance, with no major risks. An unstable patient should, of course, remain where he or she is.

1.5.2 Operation

1.5.2.1 Preoperative Preparation and Proximal Control

The management of patients with major external bleeding is mostly related to penetrating injuries to the carotid artery. Surgical exposure of this artery is described in the Technical Tips box. It is important to prepare and drape the patient for possible median sternotomy, which might be necessary to obtain proximal control. Bleeding can usually be controlled by external compression by a gloved finger during the preparation and until the complete surgical team is at hand. In the rare and challenging circumstance in which this is impossible, a nonspecialist surgeon might be forced to attempt exposure and control of the artery proximal to the injury through a separate incision with continued external finger compression over the lesion by an assistant. During control by direct finger compression of the artery, care must be taken to minimize manipulation because of the risk of thrombus fragmentation and embolization. Compression also needs to be balanced with the desire to maintain flow in the artery. Clamping the common or internal carotid artery for control might be necessary but should be avoided unless the patient's condition is life-threatening. The reason for this is the risk of embolization and cerebral ischemia due to interrupted flow. Inserting a shunt may be the only way to avoid a major stroke; the risk of major stroke in this patient category after carotid clamping may be as high as 50%. Shunting usually requires proximal and distal control, arteriotomy, and possibly also extraction of the thrombus before inserting the shunt. Extracting a thrombus requires a delicate technique and special consideration because it can easily be fragmented and dislodged as embolic masses. The safest way is to use traction with forceps and/or suction. If the extraction is followed by brisk backflow, the result is satisfactory. The use of throm-

bectomy catheters is not recommended because of the risks of mechanical disruption of the thrombus and bringing fragments up into the circle of Willis. Clamping of the external carotid artery is, on the other hand, almost always safe and can be used more liberally.

> **TECHNICAL TIPS**
> **Surgical Exposure of the Carotid Arteries**
>
> An incision anterior and parallel to the anterior border of the sternocleidomastoid muscle is recommended (Fig. 1.3). The incision can be extended dorsal to the ear and down to the sternal notch. As previously noted, preparations need to have been made to allow elongation of the incision into a median sternotomy in order to obtain proximal control of, for instance, the brachiocephalic trunk on the right side or the common carotid on the left. After the skin has been incised, subcutaneous fat is divided and, if needed, the external jugular vein ligated and divided. The sternocleidomastoid muscle is retracted posteriorly, and a dissection plane anterior to the muscle is identified. The next structure to identify is usually the facial vein and its confluence to the internal jugular vein. The former is suture-ligated and divided and is usually a very good landmark because it is located just above the carotid bifurcation. Dividing this vein allows posterior retraction of the internal jugular vein and exposure of the common carotid and its bifurcation. When preparing the carotid arteries, extreme care must be taken to avoid squeezing of the vessel, and other types of operative manipulation or trauma because of the risk of embolization to the brain. Vessel loops are applied, and the most cranial clamp is applied first to avoid embolization when the more proximal parts are clamped. Important structures to protect are the hypoglossal and vagus nerves. The former usually crosses over the internal carotid artery 2–3 cm cranial to the bifurcation and is best exposed after cranial retraction of the digastric muscle. The latter runs parallel and dorsal to the common carotid artery. The cervical ansa, often located obliquely over the carotid bifurcation, can be divided to facilitate exposure.

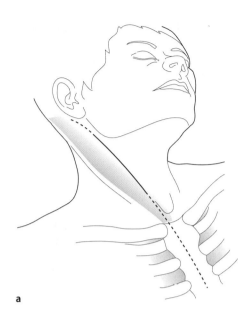

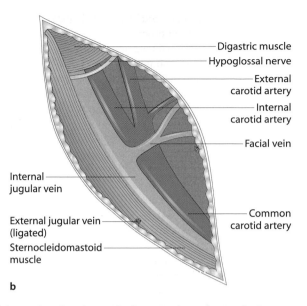

Digastric muscle
Hypoglossal nerve
External carotid artery
Internal carotid artery
Facial vein

Internal jugular vein

External jugular vein (ligated)
Sternocleidomastoid muscle

Common carotid artery

a   **b**

Fig. 1.3 a Recommended incision for exposure of the carotid arteries, anterior and parallel to the anterior border of the sternocleidomastoid muscle. The incision can be extended into a median sternotomy or cranially

dorsal to the ear. **b** The normal anatomy and relations between major arteries, veins, and important nerve structures at exposure of the carotid and jugular vessels

1.5.2.2 Exposure and Repair

For larger arterial injuries, proximal and distal control is mandatory. This always requires an indirect assessment of the cerebral perfusion by checking the backflow from the internal carotid artery. Measuring the stump pressure in the internal carotid artery is recommended if there is sufficient time. This is obtained by first clamping the common and external carotid arteries and then puncturing the internal carotid artery with a small-caliber injection needle connected to a catheter filled with saline and a pressure transducer. If the backflow is poor or the mean stump pressure is <50 mmHg, shunting is probably necessary.

Different repair techniques include the following:

- Simple suture: Simple sutures are mostly sufficient in minor penetrating injuries or small pseudoaneurysms.
- Patch: A patch can be used for a minor wall defect or to compensate for diameter loss after arteriotomy and intimal repair.

- Resection with end-to-end anastomosis: This is possible in limited injuries requiring minor resections, allowing an anastomosis without any tension.
- Resection with an interposition graft: When larger segments must be excised because of the injury, continuity might be restored with an autologous vein graft harvested from the greater saphenous vein or with prosthetic grafts for uncontaminated wounds.
- Transposition of external to internal carotid artery: This is a good alternative in special cases in which vein grafts are unavailable.
- Ligation or balloon occlusion: Ligation should be reserved for inaccessible injuries that are impossible to repair. In cases with very distal injuries to the internal carotid artery, even ligation might be difficult. An occluding balloon catheter can then be inserted into the artery at the base of the skull and insufflated until bleeding stops. The balloon catheter can be left in place for 1 to 2 days or more and then be deflated and removed.

1.5.2.3 Exploration of Minor Injuries and Hematomas

A patient with an injury penetrating the platysma in anatomical zone II without a history of bleeding may be explored by extending the traumatic skin wound to allow inspection of the injured area, including vessels, trachea, and esophagus. If, however, duplex ultrasound or angiography excludes a major vascular injury, there is no vascular indication for exploration. Patients with a history of significant bleeding as well as those with large hematomas should be treated according to what has been described above for proximal control, before exploring the wound and evacuating the hematoma.

1.5.2.4 Injuries to the Vertebral Artery

Due to its relatively inaccessible location, injuries to the vertebral artery in the cervical region are usually best treated by modern endovascular techniques. The options are intraluminal covered stents or endovascular embolization with coil. Besides bleeding and hematomas, pseudoaneurysms and arteriovenous fistulas can occur after vertebral artery trauma and also be successfully treated by transcatheter embolization. In unstable patients with life-threatening bleeding, immediate intervention with proximal and distal ligation might be necessary.

1.5.2.5 Venous Injury

Major venous injuries in the neck are almost exclusively seen after penetrating trauma. The most commonly injured veins are the external and internal jugular. Due to the low pressure in veins, many such injuries are never recognized. Isolated venous injuries consequently rarely need exploration or repair. Venous injuries encountered during exploration of a neck injury can be treated either by repair using simple or running sutures or by ligation. In bilateral injuries to the internal jugular veins, however, reconstruction of one of the sides is indicated to avoid severe venous hypertension. As in all other types of venous surgery, gentle and meticulous technique must be applied and caution taken not to extend the injuries to the veins by a traumatic technique. (See Chapter 15 on vascular surgical technique.)

1.5.2.6 Endovascular Treatment

As already described in sections 1.5.2.2 and 1.5.2.4, endovascular technique is an alternative to consider in some cervical vascular injuries. Endovascular treatment is the first option in injuries to the vertebral artery due to its location and surgical inaccessibility. The application of detachable balloons, coils, stents, or hemostatic agents is usually successful for managing bleeding, aneurysms, and fistulas. Endovascular techniques have also been reported to be successful for managing some carotid artery injuries (such as traumatic lacerations), pseudoaneurysms, and injuries in some noncritical and small terminal branches. If endovascular occlusion of an internal carotid artery is considered in severe traumatic injuries, the neurologic effect of a temporary occlusion should be evaluated prior to occlusion. It is reasonable to believe that the endovascular treatment option will become even more useful in the near future.

1.5.3 Management After Treatment

As in elective carotid surgery, monitoring and correcting blood pressure is important to minimize risks for bleeding and cerebral complications. Most common are thrombosis and reperfusion problems. Acceptable postoperative systolic blood pressure limits are 100–180 mmHg.

The patient should be checked for clinical signs and symptoms of embolization, and if embolization is suspected, the operated artery should be checked with ultrasound for complications that might need urgent repair.

Antiplatelet and/or anticoagulation therapy should be considered to maintain patency in reconstructed arteries and to avoid thrombosis in bluntly injured but still patent vessels.

Traumatic and surgical wounds should be checked for signs of a developing hematoma and infection. The latter is particularly important in contaminated wounds and when repair has included the use of prosthetic material. Antibiotic treatment should be given liberally to avoid the development of severe deep infections in penetrating cervical injuries. For the same reason, meticulous wound care is important.

Table 1.4. Stroke and mortality rates after different grades of blunt carotid and vertebral artery injuries. (From Biffl et al. Ann Surg 2002; 235: 699–707)

Injury grade/description		Carotid artery injury		Vertebral artery injury	
		Stroke	Death	Stroke	Death
I	Luminal irregularity or dissection, <25% narrowing	3%	11%	19%	31%
II	Dissection or intramural hematoma, >25% narrowing or intraluminal thrombus or raised intimal flap	11%	11%	40%	0
III	Pseudoaneurysm	33%	11%	13%	13%
IV	Occlusion	44%	22%	33%	11%
V	Transection and free extravasation	100%	100%	–	–

1.5.4 Results and Outcome

Several authors report better results after repair of penetrating injuries to the carotid artery compared with ligation, with regard to neurological outcome (44% vs. 16% neurologically intact) and mortality (5% vs. 11%).

The results of conservative treatment of carotid dissection, the most common type of injury after blunt trauma, are generally good with duplex-verified resorption of intramural hematoma within 3 months of anticoagulation. The key to this is early detection, preferably before the onset of symptoms, and institution of a heparin infusion followed by oral anticoagulation for at least 3 months. Table 1.4 above summarizes the experience of Biffl and colleagues at Brown Medical School (Rhode Island Hospital, Providence, RI, USA) from 109-patients with carotid injuries.

Recent series report good results in managing cervical vascular injuries, irrespective of zone, with only careful physical examination, but the general impression is that it is too early to eliminate angiography and duplex ultrasound from the work-up.

As seen, there is a correlation between the incidence of stroke and mortality in carotid injuries that is not found in injuries to the vertebral artery and the posterior circulation. Overall mortality after vertebral artery injuries seems to be around 20%, but this is usually in patients with a combination of other major injuries. Mortality directly related to vertebral artery injuries has been reported to be as low as 4%.

Further Reading

Baumgartner RW, Arnold M, Baumgartner I, et al. Carotid dissection with and without ischemic events; local symptoms and cerebral artery findings. Neurology 2001; 57:827–832

Biffl WL, Ray CE, Moore EE, et al. Treatment related outcomes from blunt cerebrovascular injuries. Ann Surg 2002; 235:699–707

Demetriades D, Theodorou D, Ascentio J. Management options in vertebral artery injuries. Br J Surg 1996; 83:83–86

Demetriades D, Theodoru D, Cornwell E, et al. Evaluation of penetrating injuries to the neck: prospective study of 223 patients. World J Surg 1997; 21:41–48

Gomez CR, May K, Terry J B, et al. Endovascular therapy of traumatic injuries of the extracranial cerebral arteries. Crit Care Clin 1999; 15:789–809

Kreker C, Mosso M, Georgiadis D, et al. Carotid dissection with permanent and transient occlusion or severe stenosis: long term outcome. Neurology 2003; 28:271–275

Mwipatayi BP, Jeffery P, Beningfield SJ, et al. Management of extra-cranial vertebral artery injuries. Eur J Vasc Endovasc Surg 2004; 27:157–162

Navsaria P, Omoshoro-Jones J. An analysis of 32 surgically managed penetrating carotid artery injuries. Eur J Vasc Endovasc Surg 2002; 24:349–355

Reid J, Weigfelt J. Forty-three cases of vertebral artery trauma. J Trauma 1988; 28:1007–1012

Romily RC, Newell DW, Grady MS, et al. Gunshot wounds of the internal carotid artery at the skull base: management with vein bypass grafts and a review of the literature. J Vasc Surg 2001; 33:1001–1007

Sekharan J, Dennis JW, Veldenz H, et al. Continued experience with physical examination alone for evaluation of penetrating zone 2 neck injuries; result of 145 cases. J Vasc Surg 2000; 32:483

Singh RR, Barry MC, Ireland A, et al. Current diagnosis and management of blunt internal carotid artery injury. Eur J Vasc Endovasc Surg 2004; 27:577–584

Vascular Injuries to the Thoracic Outlet Area

2

CONTENTS

2.1 Summary

- Always exclude injuries to the great thoracic aortic branches after injury to the cervical, clavikular and thoracic regions
- One third of patients who survive thoracic vascular trauma has minor or lack external signs of thoracic injury.
- A plain chest X-ray shall be performed in all patients with thoracic injuries
- Moderate restoration of BP to 100–120 mmHg is advisable to avoid rebleeding
- Be liberal with insertion of a chest tube in patients with moderate or severe hemothorax

2.2 Background

This chapter is focused on injuries to the intrathoracic parts of the great aortic branches, from their origin in the aortic arch to the thoracic outlet. It also includes the retroclavicular vessels – the distal subclavian and the proximal axillary arteries. These injuries are often difficult to diagnose and distinguish from aortic arch injuries (i.e., injuries to the aorta, the pulmonary vessels, and the heart itself). Because cardiothoracic surgeons and not vascular surgeons usually manage the latter, they will not be covered here.

A vascular injury to this region of the body is less common but is associated with high mortality. Many patients die at the scene of the accident or are in extremely bad condition at arrival in the emergency department. Accordingly, they regularly require immediate thoracotomy, but many patients are stable and possible to work up and can be treated without surgery. Most hospitals do not have a thoracic surgeon on call; therefore, these patients are often initially managed by general surgeons with limited experience in thoracic or vascular surgical procedures. Basic information about exposure and access routes and ways to achieve proximal and distal control of intrathoracic great vessels is important not only in this situation but also to obtain proximal control of bleeding vessels in cervical and proximal upper extremity vascular injuries (these areas are discussed in Chapters 1 and 3). Good anatomical knowledge, including that of common variations, is critical, especially for the difficult exposures of the subclavian and axillary vessels, such as when the right subclavian artery originates directly from the aortic arch or has a common trunk with the right carotid artery.

> **NOTE**
> Anatomical aortic arch and branch variations can be expected in 25–35% of cases.

2.2.1 Magnitude of the Problem

The number of thoracic injuries (all types included) is steadily increasing in the United States and is estimated to be 12 per million inhabitants per year. In penetrating neck and chest injuries, 3% are associated with injuries to the subclavian and axillary arteries, and in 20% of those injuries, veins are also injured. In a meta-analysis of 2,642 civilian cases of penetrating thoracic trauma, the incidence of great vessel injuries was 1% innominate artery, 5% subclavian, and 6% axillary artery injuries. But because many patients die at the scene, particularly after penetrating trauma, these numbers are uncertain. Irrespective of the type of injuries, trauma to the thoracic great vessels is associated with a high mortality: 80–90% die at the scene. The mortality among patients who survive transport to the hospital is also high.

Patients with injuries in the distal parts of the intrathoracic arteries have a better chance of survival because these vessels are covered with soft tissue, providing better prerequisites for spontaneous tamponade.

More proximal injuries increase the risk for exsanguination into the pleural cavities. Venous injuries often remain unrecognized. Arteriograms in patients with a widened mediastinum on plain x-ray after thoracic trauma have been found to be negative for arterial injuries in 85%; this suggests that the mediastinal enlargement was caused mainly by venous injury.

> **NOTE**
> Injuries to subclavian and axillary arteries are most common after penetrating trauma.

2.2.2 Etiology and Pathophysiology

2.2.2.1 Penetrating Trauma

Knife stabbings or missiles from firearms cause a majority of injuries to the great vessels. In this type of penetrating trauma, all intrathoracic vessels are at risk of being injured. The extent of injuries is related to aspects of the weapon, such as the length of a knife or the velocity (high vs. low) and caliber (small vs. large) of a gun. The innominate artery is injured mostly by bullets from firearms. Stab wounds by knives directed inferiorly into the right clavicular region may also damage the innominate artery. The same mechanisms are common for injuries to the subclavian and proximal axillary arteries. Stab wounds are associated with a better chance of survival than are injuries from firearms, particularly shotguns. Blood loss after a knife injury is often limited by a sealing mechanism in the wound channel. Furthermore, if the vascular injury is small, the adventitia also limits the bleeding.

The development of hypotension is another factor contributing to limited blood loss. Injuries to the major blood vessels in the thoracic outlet are always challenging because they are rare and technically difficult to expose and control. This is reflected in the high mortality reported in the literature.

2.2.2.2 Blunt Trauma

Blunt trauma to the intrathoracic vessels occurs in motor vehicle and industrial accidents and in falls from heights. If it leads to total disruption of the vessel, the patient will exsanguinate at the scene. When the adventitia remains intact, the possibility of survival is better. The mechanism is shear caused by acceleration/deceleration or compression forces. Deceleration forces are associated with injuries to the aorta but may also cause injuries to the innominate artery. The innominate and common carotid artery might be exposed to shear forces at their origin from compression of the anterior chest wall. The subclavian and axillary arteries can also be injured by blunt trauma, and then mostly in association with clavicle or 1st-rib fractures. Other possible mechanisms are hyperextension combined with neck rotation, causing tension and stretching of the contralateral subclavian vessels. Alternative mechanisms include stretching over the clavicle. Blunt injuries to the subclavian artery after deceleration trauma are rare. There are, however, some controversies regarding the association between 1st-rib fractures and injuries to the subclavian vessels. Two series of 49 and 55 patients, respectively, reported an incidence of 14% and 5% of vascular injuries in association with rib fractures. On the other hand, in a large cohort of 466 patients only 0.4% was found.

NOTE

Injuries to large veins in the thoracic outlet region are associated with a risk of air embolism and if this occurs, it significantly increases mortality.

2.3 Clinical Presentation

2.3.1 Medical History

The diagnosis is obvious in most cases of penetrating vascular trauma, but the following information is important for management. In injuries caused by a firearm, the type of weapon used (shotgun, hand weapon, high or low velocity, small or large caliber) and the distance from where it was fired are relevant. For knife stabbings, the blade length and size are important, as well as the angle and direction in which it struck the body. Stabbings directed inferiorly in the clavicular region or at the base of the neck are associated with an increased risk for injuries to the innominate or subclavian arteries.

In blunt trauma, information about the direction and localization of force, the velocity of the motor vehicle, use of a safety belt, or the height of a fall can indicate the risk for intrathoracic vascular injuries.

When deciding whether immediate thoracotomy is needed, the course of transport and time elapsed from injury to admission is always of potential importance.

2.3.2 Clinical Signs

As in other vascular injuries, the following "hard signs" strongly indicate severe vascular injury:
- Severe bleeding
- Shock or severe anemia
- Expanding hematoma
- Absent or weak peripheral pulses
- Bruits

"Soft signs" that also indicate vascular injuries include the following:
- Local and stable hematoma
- Minor continuous bleeding
- Mild hypotension
- Proximity to large vessels
- Any periclavicular trauma

Injuries to the large vessels in the thorax are frequently associated with injuries to the aerodigestive tract. The following signs and symptoms should alert the responsible surgeon to exclude underlying severe vascular injuries:
- Air bubbles in the wound
- Respiratory distress
- Subcutaneous emphysema
- Hoarseness
- Hemoptysis
- Hematemesis

NOTE

Patients with periclavicular trauma should always be suspected to have intrathoracic great vessel injuries.

Intrathoracic injuries to the subclavian and axillary arteries are associated with high mortality. Like injuries to the thoracic aorta, the presentation varies widely, from a fairly stable to a more extreme situation with massive bleeding and exsanguination and death at the scene or during transport. The latter is more common after blunt trauma that causes avulsion of great vessels and penetrating trauma to the subclavian artery or vein. The consequence of subclavian vessel injury is bleeding into the pleural cavity with or without air embolization. At arrival in the emergency department, a patient with a penetrating intrathoracic vascular injury is typically hemodynamically unstable, whereas a blunt vessel injury is not always immediately apparent.

Blunt injuries to the innominate artery are relatively rare, and 75% are combined with other injuries such as rib fractures, flail chest, hemothorax or pneumothorax, extremity or facial fractures, or head or abdominal injuries in multitrauma cases. Because there are no typical clinical signs or symptoms, diagnosis is difficult. The only frequent clinical finding is that 50–70% of such patients have a weak radial or brachial pulse. Distal extremity ischemia is uncommon, however, due to good collateral circulation in the shoulder region. This explains the possibility of having a palpable distal pulse despite a severe proximal arterial injury.

The subclavian artery is usually injured by direct trauma associated with first-rib or clavicular fractures that cause occlusion of the artery. About half of the patients have a combined injury to the brachial plexus. Accordingly, clinical signs and symptoms indicating such neurological injuries (see Chapter 3, p. 33) should increase the suspicion of injuries associated with the subclavian artery.

2.3.2.1 Physical Examination

The entire thorax should be inspected for stab wounds. It is important not to forget skin folds, the axilla, or areas with thick hair. A penetrating trauma to this region is always obvious at arrival in the emergency department. It is also important to remember that one-third of patients who survive blunt trauma and are taken to the emergency department have minor or even no external signs of thoracic injury.

A pulsatile mass or hematoma at the base of the neck, with or without a bruit, indicates an injury to the subclavian artery with leakage through the vessel wall.

At physical examination, auscultation can reveal signs of hemothorax or pneumothorax. The entire chest and back should be auscultated for bruits. A systolic bruit over the back and upper chest usually indicates a false aneurysm in any of the great intrathoracic vessels. A continuous bruit indicates the presence of an arteriovenous fistula.

Peripheral pulses, including axillary, brachial, and radial, should always be examined. They are normal in about half of cases with significant vessel injury. Absence of a radial pulse indicates a injury to the axillary, subclavian, or innominate arteries, causing occlusion, dissection, or embolization. The latter is occasionally caused by an embolizing bullet.

A thorough neurological evaluation is also relevant when considering the possibility of combined brachial plexus and vascular injuries. The absence of a radial pulse in combination with Horner's syndrome is suspicious for injury to the subclavian artery.

Coma or major neurological deficits can also occur as a consequence of injuries to the innominate and common carotid arteries leading to occlusion or embolization and different levels of cerebral ischemia. Therefore, it is important to evaluate the patient's mental status upon admission. The result influences the decision about if and when to perform emergency surgical repair. This evaluation may also be important during the course of management as a baseline for later reevaluations.

The management and diagnostic work-up in the emergency department are strongly related to the condition in which the patient arrives. In these types of injuries, the patient is often in an extreme condition, requiring immediate transfer to the operating room for an emergency thoracotomy or other surgical repair. Thoracotomy may even be indicated in the emergency department for a dying patient.

NOTE

One-third of patients who survive blunt thoracic vascular trauma have minor or no external signs of thoracic injury.

2.4 Diagnostics

At arrival, most patients are in a condition that necessitates immediate transfer to the operating room for surgical exploration and treatment. In the remaining patients, the diagnostic work-up depends on the type of trauma and the patient's condition. In a stable patient, such examinations can provide information of great importance for the management strategy. A good rule is not to start time-consuming examinations while the patient is still hemodynamically unstable.

In a stable patient, plain neck and chest x-rays should always be done to see whether he or she has any of the following:

- Hemothorax or pneumothorax
- Widened mediastinum
- Irregular outline of the descending aorta
- Tracheal dislocation
- Blurring of the aortic knob
- Dilatation of the aortic bulb
- Presence of bullets or fracture fragments
- Fractures in cervical vertebrae, clavicles, or ribs

Duplex examination has its limitations for detecting injuries to the innominate and subclavian arteries because of their deep intrathoracic location, particularly in obese patients. It is also examiner-dependent, but nowadays a first choice in many centers. Transesophageal echocardiography may be valuable for diagnosing aortic injuries, but less so in injuries to the aortic branches.

Spiral computed tomography (CT) with intravenous contrast is mostly used to obtain information about a missile's direction and trajectory through the body. The trajectory's vicinity to great vessels is important when selecting patients for angiography. The modern multislice CT angiography has the potential to become an important diagnostic tool for providing more detailed description of thoracic vascular injuries.

Angiography can be diagnostic as well as therapeutic. It reveals the presence and localization of occlusions, bleeding, leakage, or pseudoaneurysms as well as intimal tears. To detect potential tears and other injuries in the innominate artery, aortography should be performed with posterior oblique projections. A bulbous dilatation at or just distal to its origin and the visualization of an intimal flap in the lumen indicate a tear injury to the artery.

In subclavian injuries, a pseudoaneurysm or occlusion can be found. It is important to remember that 10% of patients with innominate or subclavian injuries also have other injuries to great

intrathoracic vessels, why it is important that the angiography visualizes the entire thoracic aorta and its branches. The endovascular treatment of these injuries is discussed later in this chapter.

Chest tube placement should have liberal indications for diagnostic as well as therapeutic purposes, as a chest tube can reveal the presence of hemothorax or pneumothorax. The technique is described in detail in the section on management below.

NOTE
A plain chest x-ray should be performed in all patients with thoracic trauma.

2.5 Management and Treatment

2.5.1 Management Before Treatment

2.5.1.1 Management in the Emergency Department

Management of these often severely injured patients in shock follows the usual Advanced Trauma Life Support principles of trauma resuscitation. The first priority is always airway control and resuscitation for hypovolemia. Injuries to the great vessels in the thoracic outlet frequently result in expanding mediastinal hematoma, causing tracheal compression and requiring emergency endotracheal intubation.

1. Clear and maintain the airway.
2. Secure ventilation by endotracheal intubation and 100% oxygen.
3. Consider chest tube insertion.
4. Place two or three intravenous lines, preferably in the legs and/or the opposite arm.
5. Support adequate circulation by rapid volume replacement with 2.000–3.000 ml of a warm balanced electrolyte solution and blood products.
6. Control bleeding. (See below.)
7. Consider putting the patient in Trendelenburg position to avoid air embolism when major venous injuries cannot be excluded.
8. Insert a Foley catheter.

As in patients with a ruptured abdominal aortic aneurysm, resuscitation aims at keeping blood pressure around 100–120-mmHg because of the risk of sudden massive rebleeding if the blood pressure gets too high. Another event posing risk for new bleeding during resuscitation is gagging during endotracheal intubation or the insertion of an esophageal tube.

If possible, obtain written consent from the patient or his or her family in case emergency surgery is necessary. The surgical procedure that may be required often includes clamping of central arteries, the aorta, or the common carotids, with a great risk for severe cerebral and spinal complications. Therefore, it is advisable to alert an experienced thoracic and/or vascular surgeon for early help with management.

NOTE
Moderate restoration of blood pressure to 100–120 mmHg is advisable to avoid rebleeding.

2.5.1.2 Patients in Extreme Shock

In this category are patients who, most commonly after penetrating thoracic trauma, have lost consciousness and present with no vital signs despite resuscitation during the transport but who still show activity on electrocardiography. Other patients in this category are those with acute therapy-resistant deterioration, those with severe and persistent shock despite very rapid and aggressive volume resuscitation (2.000–3.000 ml of fluids within minutes) and systolic blood pressure <50 mmHg, and those who experience cardiac arrest in the emergency department. These patients are candidates for thoracotomy in the emergency department, aiming at controlling bleeding by manual compression, tamponade, or clamping. This allows more effective resuscitation and is a last lifesaving effort to improve these patients' vital functions enough to allow transfer to the operating room for immediate surgery.

In such an extreme situation, surgeons with no or only limited experience in thoracotomy can be forced to choose between the two ultimate alternatives: to open the patient's chest or to let him or her die. The prognosis for such a patient is, irrespective of who is performing the thoracotomy, poor, and the survival rate is only around 5%. This should be weighed against the alternative, which is 100% mortality. More than 20% of patients with injuries to subclavian and axillary vessels are in an extreme condition with no vital signs or with imminent cardiac rest upon arrival to the emergency department. These patients have a very poor prognosis.

NOTE
Do not hesitate to perform a thoracotomy in the emergency department on a patient with persistent electrocardiographic activity but with no detectable vital signs.

TECHNICAL TIPS
Chest Tube Insertion

Start by determining the desired site of insertion. The recommended site is the 4th or 5th intercostal space, landmark the nipple level just anterior to the midaxillary line, which is good for draining air as well as blood. Scrub and drape the predetermined area. Anesthetize the skin, intercostal muscles, pleura, and rib periosteum locally (Fig. 2.1 a).

Make a 3 to 4 cm long skin incision over the intercostal space, parallel to the ribs (Fig. 2.1 b). Bluntly dissect the subcutaneous tissue over the cranial aspect of the rib to avoid the intercostal vessels. Continue dissection down to the pleura, preferably with a curved clamp or a finger. Then puncture the parietal pleura with the tip of a clamp and then expand it with a gloved finger. This is to take precautions against iatrogenic injury to the lung (Fig. 2.1 c, d).

Insert a catheter (32-French or 36-French) with the curved clamp and guide it with a finger. To drain blood, it is best to direct it posterolaterally, and to remove air, an apical position is preferred.

Correct intrapleural position is indicated by "fogging" in the catheter during respiration and when the first side hole is 1 to 2 cm inside the chest wall. Connect the tube to a water-suction device. Secure the tube with a separate suture, and suture the skin.

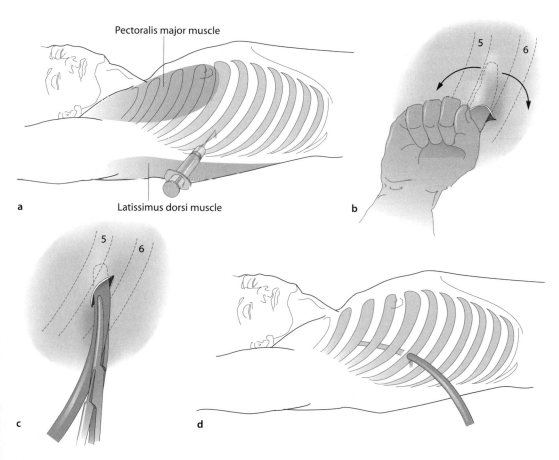

Fig. 2.1. Steps for chest tube insertion

TECHNICAL TIPS
Emergency Anterolateral 5th-Interspace Thoracotomy for Control of the Aorta

The patient must be intubated and ventilated. Incise the skin from the sternum to the axillary line along the upper border of the 5th rib on the left side. In women, the submamillary groove is a landmark. Continue cutting the muscles with scissors or a scalpel all the way down to the pleura. Open the pleural sheath with a pair of scissors. The opening should be as large as the hand. One or two costal cartilages can be cut to obtain better access through the thoracotomy. Follow the aortic arch, pass the left subclavian artery and pulmonary artery, and mobilize the heart slightly to the right. Press the descending aorta manually or with an aortic occluder against the spine and try to achieve the best possible occlusion. This occlusion is maintained under continuous fluid resuscitation and while the patient is transferred to the operating room. Alternatively, place a Satinsky clamp just distal to the origin of the left subclavian artery. The proximal blood pressure must be kept <180 mmHg after clamp placement, and it should be removed as soon as possible.

The left subclavian artery is, in contrast to the right, an intrapleural structure and can in most cases be visualized relatively easy and directly compressed with a finger, clamped, or packed. A left-sided thoracotomy can be extended over to the right, aiming at a higher interstitium. If, however, it is obvious that the injury is on the right side, the thoracotomy should be performed on that side. Severe right-sided intrathoracic bleeding is best controlled by finger compression and packing a tamponade in the apex of the right pleural cavity, combined with heavy manual compression in the right supraclavicular fossa.

If resuscitation fails despite adequate fluid substitution and successful control of bleeding, air embolism should be suspected if there are injuries to large veins. Puncture and aspiration in the right ventricle is diagnostic as well as therapeutic.

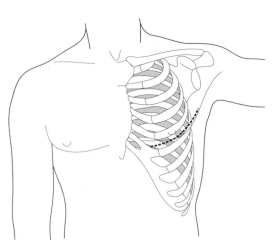

Fig. 2.2. Incision for emergency anterolateral thoracotomy

2.5.1.3 Unstable Patients

Patients with blood pressure <50 mmHg and in severe shock are candidates for immediate surgery. A rapid infusion of 2–3 l of a balanced electrolyte solution over 10–15 min should be given, aiming to keep blood pressure between 70 and 90 mmHg. It is probably important to keep this level of blood pressure to avoid the risk of increased bleeding associated with a higher blood pressure. If the patient does not respond to this volume replacement, he or she should be taken to the operating room for immediate surgery.

Antibiotics covering staphylococci and streptococci should be administered according to the local protocols. One suggestion is cephalosporins. Analgesics, morphine 10 mg intravenously, and, in penetrating injuries, prophylaxis against tetanus should also be administered.

2.5.1.4 Control of Bleeding

In penetrating injuries with continued external bleeding, control is achieved by finger compression over the wound. A gloved finger can also be inserted into the wound to compress the bleeding and stop the outflow of blood. Another recommended method is to insert a 24-French Foley catheter into the wound tract and fill the balloon with water or saline (Fig. 2.3). The catheter is clamped after insufflation of the balloon, and if

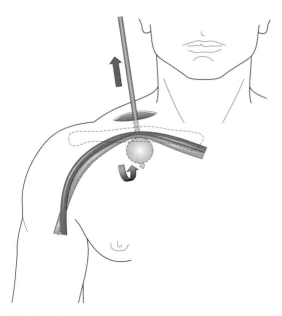

Fig. 2.3. Temporary balloon tamponade of bleeding after penetrating injury to a major subclavian vessel. A Foley catheter is gently inserted to the bottom of the wound tract. After the balloon is filled with saline, gentle traction is applied to the catheter, causing compression of the vessels against the clavicle

the wound penetrates into the pleural cavity, it is gently pulled so the balloon tamponades the pleural entrance. If external bleeding persists after this maneuver, a second balloon can be inserted into the wound and insufflated to stop external bleeding from the wound tract. By applying some traction to the catheters, the balloon can also compress injured vessels against the clavicle or the ribs.

If there are clinical indications or radiological signs of moderate or large hemothorax, a chest tube should be inserted for its evacuation. The rationale is that a hemothorax can contribute to continued intrathoracic bleeding and restrict ventilation and venous return. Depending on the results when the pleural cavity is drained, different actions can be taken. In an unstable patient, the following are considered strong indicators for emergency thoracotomy:

- 1.500 ml of blood drained directly after insertion of the tube

- >300 ml blood drained through the tube within an hour
- Deterioration of vital signs when the drain is opened

Even in initially unstable patients, this strategy with evacuation of hemothorax and volume replacement is often successful. It may allow enough time to let the patient undergo emergency work-up under close surveillance. Information obtained from CT scanning and/or angiography facilitates decisions regarding optimal positioning and routes for exposure of the injury at final surgical treatment (see section 2.5.2, p. 25–27). As described below, in many situations this type of management stabilizes the patient enough to allow continued nonsurgical management.

NOTE
Be liberal with chest tube insertion in patients with moderate or severe hemothorax.

2.5.1.5 Stable Patients
Initial management is the same as described above for unstable patients or patients in extreme shock, as summarized in Table 2.1.

Diagnostic examinations in stable patients include repeat plain chest x-ray, angiography or duplex ultrasound under close surveillance. Also in stable patients chest tubes should be placed on liberal indications for evacuation and monitoring of bleeding. The following indicate continued bleeding and the possible need for surgical treatment:

- Deterioration of vital signs (i.e., hypotensive reaction) when the drain is started
- 1.500–2.000 ml of blood within the first 4–8 h
- Drainage of blood exceeding 300 ml/h for more than 4 h
- More than half of pleural cavity filled with blood on x-ray despite a well functioning chest tube

All of these factors may indicate thoracotomy and should alert the surgeon to consider operation and contact with a cardiothoracic surgeon when needed.

Table 2.1. Initial work-up and treatment of patients with thoracic outlet vascular injuries of different severity (*US* ultrasound, *CT* computed tomography, *ED* emergency department, *OR* operating room)

Patient's condition	Responds to resuscitation	US	CT	Angiography	Treatment
Extreme shock	No	No	No	No	Emergency thoracotomy in the ED
Unstable	No	No	No	No	Emergency thoracotomy in the OR or ED
	Yes	Maybe	Maybe	Yes	As above or continued non-op management if only moderate injuries
Stable	Yes	Maybe	Maybe	Yes	Operative or nonoperative management depending on findings
	Deteriorates after opening chest drain	No	No	Maybe	Emergency operation in the OR

2.5.1.6 Nonsurgical Management

An initially unstable patient who responds well to resuscitation and becomes stable, as well as stable patients with a continued stable course, and with no major vascular injury necessitating surgery revealed at the work-up can often be managed by blood transfusions, fluid replacement, and a chest tube to drain a hemothorax.

The management of patients with major neurological deficits or coma is a matter of debate. Many physicians argue that these patients are never candidates for surgical intervention due to their severe brain injury and poor prognosis. Others argue that vascular injuries should be repaired in all of these cases because it is impossible to exclude that the unconsciousness is related to some injury other than a vascular one.

2.5.2 Operation

2.5.2.1 Preoperative Preparation and Proximal Control

The patient is scrubbed and draped to allow incisions from the neck down to at least the knee. In an emergency situation without knowledge about the exact injury site, the patient is best positioned supine with the arms abducted 30°.

The aim of emergency thoracotomy in an unstable patient is primarily to control bleeding. This can be achieved by surgeons without experience in cardiothoracic surgery. Once control is accomplished, the repair can wait to allow time for further resuscitation and for experienced assistance to arrive. Most experienced trauma surgeons today recommend a median sternotomy because it is considered the most versatile approach. Such an incision can easily be extended up along the sternocleidomastoid muscle on either side or laterally over the clavicle as needed. This approach is therefore recommended when localization of the injury is uncertain (Fig. 2.4).

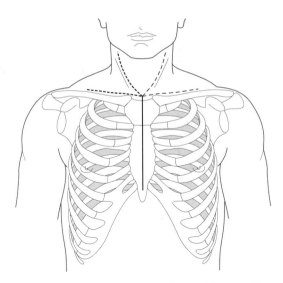

Fig. 2.4. Median sternotomy with possible extensions for proximal and distal control in vascular injuries in the thoracic outlet region

2.5.2.2 Exposure and Repair

For innominate artery injuries, the median sternotomy is extended along the anterior border of the sternocleidomastoid muscle to the right. The overlying innominate vein, which is often also injured, has to be divided to achieve exposure. If the injury is located at the base of the artery, which is common in blunt trauma, a reconstruction with an 8–10-mm prosthetic graft end-to-side from the ascending aorta to the divided innominate is frequently employed. This can be performed with only a partially occluding clamp on the aorta. A total exposure of the proximal aorta and the innominate bifurcation is, however, frequently needed for proximal and distal control before opening the hematoma. In minor penetrating injuries, simple sutures may occasionally be sufficient (Fig. 2.5).

The need for shunting to prevent cerebral ischemia during innominate artery clamping is controversial. Some argue that it is not needed if (1) clamping is caudal to the origin of the common carotid artery, (2) blood pressure and cardiac output are normal, and (3) the contralateral carotid artery is open. Others believe it is preferable to always measure stump pressure in the common carotid artery distal to the innominate clamp. Shunting is recommended if the mean pressure is <50 mmHg or not measurable.

Injuries to the common carotid arteries are exposed and managed according to the same guidelines as for innominate injuries. Proximal injuries can be repaired by a prosthetic bypass or simple suture. In cases with occlusion also involving the internal carotid artery, ligation is the safest method. This applies for neurologically intact patients as well as those who are in deep coma.

The subclavian arteries, in particular the retroclavicular portion of the left artery, are difficult to expose and manage. Before approaching the injured area it is extremely important to have a strategy for how to obtain proximal control in these injuries; otherwise, severe uncontrollable bleeding may occur. The subclavian arteries can be exposed

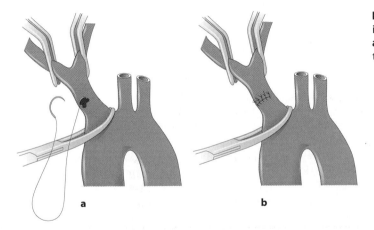

a   b

Fig. 2.5. Repair of a penetrating injury to the innominate artery. **a** Clamp occlusion at the origin from the aorta. **b** Final repair with suture

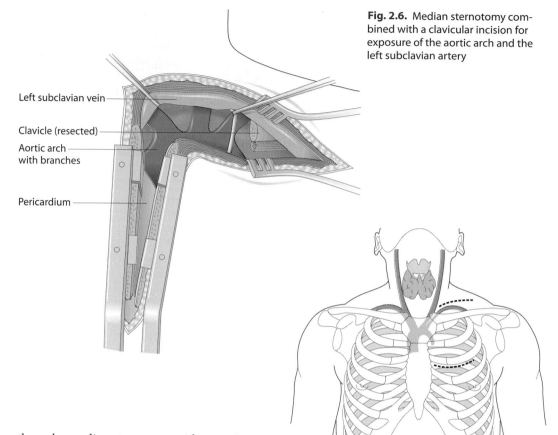

Fig. 2.6. Median sternotomy combined with a clavicular incision for exposure of the aortic arch and the left subclavian artery

Left subclavian vein

Clavicle (resected)

Aortic arch
with branches

Pericardium

through a median sternotomy with extensions supraclavicularly on the side of the injury. This route also allows exposure of injuries in the proximal left subclavian artery (Fig. 2.6).

On the left side, an alternative for proximal control is a high thoracotomy in the 3rd intercostal space combined with a supraclavicular incision for distal control (Fig. 2.7).

A thoracotomy is not necessary in injuries to the distal subclavian and proximal axillary artery. The recommended approach for control in these cases is a clavicular incision, starting at the sternoclavicular joint, extending over the medial portion of the clavicle to curve down into the deltopectoral groove. The exposure of the retroclavicular portion of the subclavian artery sometimes requires division of the major pectoral and subclavian muscles, the sternoclavicular joint, and the clavicle. After these procedures, the medial portion of the clavicle can be resected or rotated laterally. Clavicular resection in combination can also be employed with a laterally extended median

Fig. 2.7. In unstable patients and when rapid bleeding control is needed, some prefer an anterior 3rd-interspace thoracotomy in combination with a supraclavicular incision for distal control of the subclavian artery

sternotomy. By placing a longitudinal pillow between the shoulders of the patient, the shoulder can be pushed dorsally to further facilitate exposure (Fig. 2.8).

Principles of repair of the subclavian and axillary arteries usually involve resection and interposition grafting. Autogenous vein graft is the first choice, but polytetrafluoroethylene (PTFE) or polyester grafts are alternatives. Resection and end-to-end anastomosis are rarely possible, and these vessels are particularly fragile, thus increasing the risk for tension in the anastomosis.

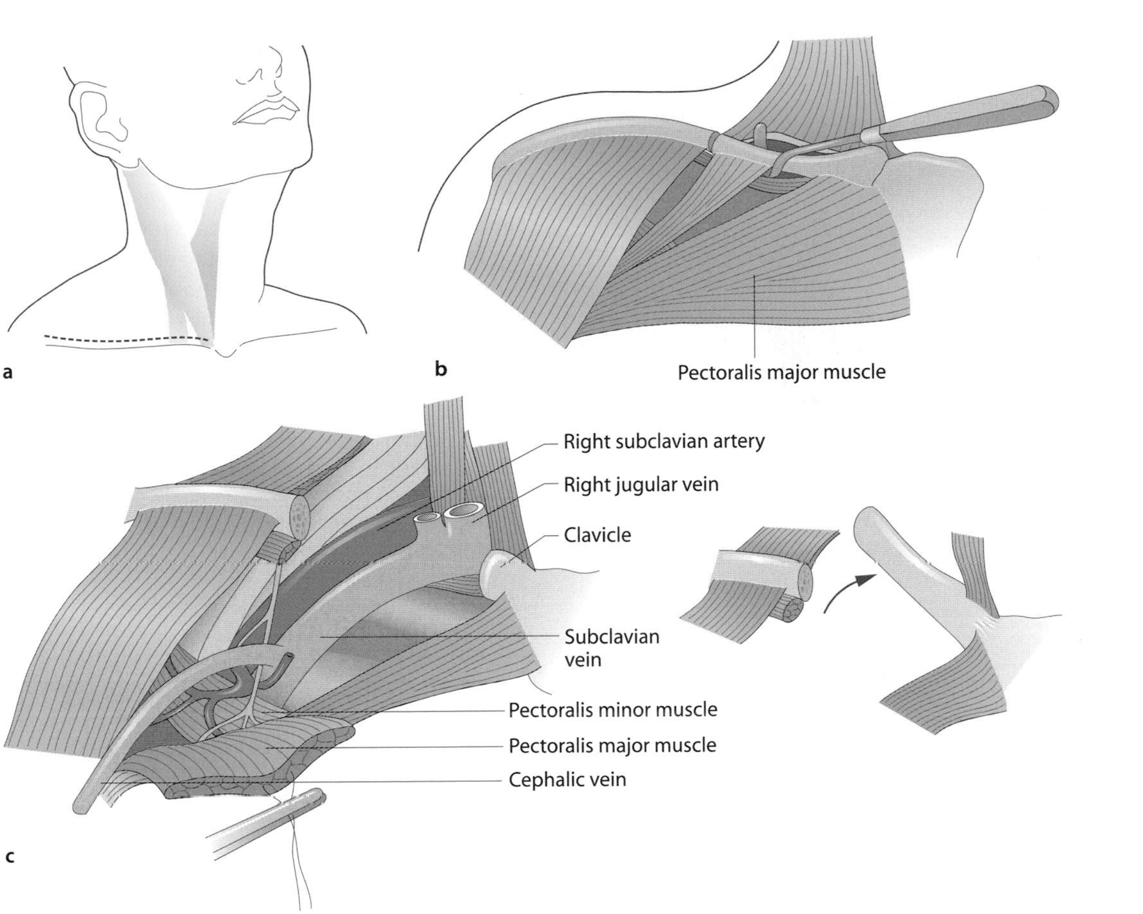

Pectoralis major muscle

Right subclavian artery

Right jugular vein

Clavicle

Subclavian vein

Pectoralis minor muscle

Pectoralis major muscle

Cephalic vein

Fig. 2.8. Exposure of the distal subclavian and proximal axillary artery. **a** A clavicular incision is used. **b** The sternocleidomastoid, pectoralis major, and subclavian muscles are stripped of the medial half of the clavicle. **c** The clavicle is divided and its medial portion resected or retracted. If necessary, the pectoralis minor muscle is divided

2.5.2.3 Endovascular Repair and Control

The use of endovascular methods in trauma management is increasing. So far, insertion of covered stents has been used successfully to seal leaks and pseudoaneurysms (Fig. 2.9).

Coils are useful for occluding bleeding branches. Another evolving management technique is to place balloon catheters in the innominate or proximal left subclavian artery for temporary proximal control. This minimally invasive endovascular alternative, when applicable, is particularly attractive in multiply injured patients by allowing time for managing other major injuries.

The vascular segments of the thoracic outlet region can be catheterized by puncturing the common femoral artery of either side or the contralateral brachial artery.

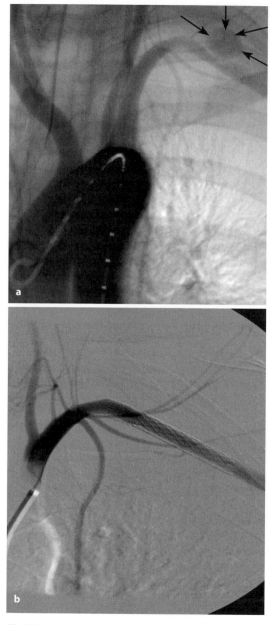

2.5.3 Management After Treatment

The proximity of the great vessels and trachea gives high priority to respiration and airways in the early postoperative period. Intubation is usually required. Many patients with injuries to the aortic arch branches require chest tubes for draining the thorax. Close monitoring of the chest tube for signs of bleeding is important because this is the most common postoperative complication. More than 300 ml of blood drained per hour is usually considered a clear indication for reexploration to exclude or repair surgical causes of the bleeding. Dilutional thrombocytopenia and hypothermia are other possible causes of postoperative bleeding problems. The recommendation is to remove the chest tube within 24 h or as soon as the risk of bleeding is considered to be under control.

Associated neurological symptoms caused by the initial trauma or the repair are common. Examples are injuries to the phrenic and vagal nerves. Secondary ischemic cerebral injuries also occur, and if aggravated during the postoperative course, this indicates embolization or thrombotic occlusion of a repaired or traumatized arterial segment.

2.6 Results

In textbooks the results are generally considered poor for patients with thoracic outlet injuries, but case series give some hope, at least for patients who reach the hospital alive.

A large series of 228 patients from South Africa with penetrating thoracic outlet vascular trauma reported that 60% of the patients were dead on admission. The operative mortality was 15% for the remaining patients, giving a total mortality of 66%. In a report from Los Angeles, the corresponding figures were a 34% total mortality and 15% operative mortality.

Fig. 2.9. a Penetrating injury to the left subclavian artery after a knife stabbing with extravasation of contrast into a pseudoaneurysm (*arrows*) at angiography. **b** No leakage after sealing the injury with a covered stent

The results, however, vary greatly between different studies. In a study from 1989 30 patients with blunt thoracic vascular trauma, substantially better results were reported; the operative mortality was 6.7%, and overall graft patency was 90% after 5 years of follow-up. Another report from the same year had a similar mortality rate of 6.5%. It included 46 patients with 51 intrathoracic arterial injuries, 42 of which were penetrating injuries. The incidence of neurological consequences in the different series was relatively low, 5–29%. Combined arterial and venous injuries or venous injuries are associated with a significantly higher mortality, up to 50% and higher. This is blamed the risk for air embolization and more severe blood loss due to less contractility of the veins.

In summary, it seems that most patients die at the scene or during transport, but if the patient arrives alive in the emergency department, the results seem to be fair.

■ Further Reading

Abouljoud MS, Obeid FN, Horst HM. Arterial injury to the thoracic outlet – a ten year experience. Am Surg 1993; 59:590–595

Axisa BM, Loftus IM, Fishwick G, et al. Endovascular repair of an innominate artery false aneurysm following blunt trauma. J Endovasc Ther 2000; 7:245–250

Cox CS, Allen GS, Fischer RP, et al. Blunt versus penetrating subclavian artery injury: Presentation, injury pattern, and outcome. J Trauma 1999; 46:445–449

Demetriades D, Chahwan S, Gomez H, et al. Penetrating injury to the subclavian and axillary vessels. J Am Coll Surg 1999; 188:290–295

Hajarizadeh H, Rohrer MJ, Cutler BS. Surgical exposure of the left subclavian artery by median sternotomy and left supraclavicular extension. J Trauma 1996; 41:136–139

Hoff SJ, Reilly MK, Merrill WH, et al. Analysis of blunt and penetrating injury of the innominate and subclavian arteries. Am Surg 1994; 60:151–154

Pate JW, Cole FH, Walker WA, et al. Penetrating injury of the aortic arch and its branches. Am Thor Surg 1993; 55:586–589

Miles EJ, Buche A, Thompson W, et al. Endovascular repair of acute innominate artery injury due to blunt trauma. Am Surg 2003; 69(2):155–159

Weiman DS, McCoy DW, Haan CK, et al. Blunt injury of the brachiocephalic artery. Am Surg 1998; 64(5):383–387

Vascular Injuries in the Arm

3

CONTENTS

■ 3.1 Summary

- Suspect vascular injuries in patients with shoulder or elbow dislocation.
- When blood pressures in the arms differ, exclude vascular injuries in proximal arteries.
- It is the nerve injury that determines the functional outcome of arm injuries.
- Evaluate the brachial plexus and the median nerve function before and during vascular exploration.
- Repair of vascular injuries in the upper limb is wise even when ischemia appears to be limited.

■ 3.2 Background

■ 3.2.1 Background

Arteries and veins in the arms are the second most common location for vessel injuries in the body and constitute almost half of all peripheral vascular injuries. Much more often than in the legs they occur together with neurological and skeletal injuries. Although vascular injuries in the arms rarely lead to fatal or serious bleeding, ischemic consequences are common. The extensive collateral network around the elbow makes clinical signs variable and often minute. On the other hand, if the brachial artery is obstructed proximal to the origin of the deep brachial artery, the risk for amputation is substantial: up to 50% of such patients lose the arm if the vessel is not repaired. While the vascular injury per se often can be managed easily, it is the damaged nerves that cause the main functional disturbances in the long run.

Because arm vessel trauma is common and sometimes appear without signs and symptoms, missed injuries cause considerable morbidity in trauma patients. Awareness and optimal management may reduce this morbidity.

The arteries supplying blood to the arms – the subclavian and axillary arteries – are located in the thorax or thoracic outlet, and if these vessels are traumatized, the consequences are often more serious. This "intrathoracic part of the arm" is covered in Chapter 2 on vascular injuries in the thoracic outlet area.

◼ 3.2.2 Etiology and Pathophysiology

Injury mechanisms are the same in the arms and legs, and the brachial, radial, and ulnar arteries can be damaged by both penetrating and blunt trauma. Knives and gunshots usually cause penetrating injuries (most often to the brachial artery), but lacerations secondary to fractures occur regularly. Sharp fragments commonly penetrate vessel walls (Fig. 3.1). Blunt injuries occur in road traffic accidents because of fractures and joint dislocations. The most frequent orthopedic arm injuries associated with vessel damage are listed in Table 3.1.

There are also types of trauma specific for arm vessel injuries. A large number of upper limb vascular trauma are caused by industrial and domestic accidents. Splintered glass as well as self-inflicted wounds regularly damage vessels below the elbow. The popularity of using the brachial artery as a site for vascular access for endovascular procedures has caused an increase in iatrogenic catheter-related injuries to the brachial artery in proximity to the elbow. Pseudoaneurysms are often caused by radial artery punctures for arterial blood samples.

As in all traumatized vessels, transection or laceration may cause bleeding, thrombosis, or both. Transections, intimal tears, and contusions are more frequent after blunt trauma. The mechanisms are described in more detail in Chapter 9 (p. 102). Tissue in the distal parts of the arm is as susceptible to ischemia as in the legs, and the time limit of 6–8 h before irreversible damage occurs is also valid for arm injuries. Concomitant nerve injuries, as mentioned, are the main cause of mor-

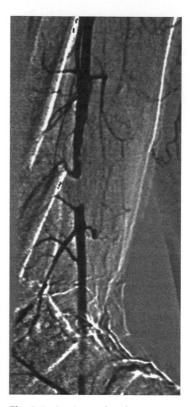

Fig. 3.1. Angiography showing an occluded brachial artery severed by the sharp ends of a shaft fracture of the humerus

Table 3.1. Most common sites for combined orthopedic and vascular injury

Orthopedic injury	Vascular injury
Fractured clavicle	Subclavian artery
Shoulder dislocation	Axillary artery
Supracondylar fracture of the humerus	Brachial artery
Elbow dislocation	Brachial artery

bidity long term. Such injuries are equally common after penetrating and blunt trauma. In the literature, 35–60% of arterial injuries in the upper arm are associated with nerve injuries, and over 75% are associated with nerve, bone, or venous damage.

3.3 Clinical Presentation

3.3.1 Medical History

Patients with vascular injuries in the arms arrive at the emergency department after accidents, knife or shooting assaults, or car crashes causing multiple injuries. As with all injuries, it is important to interview the rescue personnel and accompanying persons about the type of injury and the type of bleeding. The exact time of the injury should be established to facilitate planning of repair. Because orthopedic injuries are associated with arterial damage, it is also essential to ask whether joint dislocations or fractures were noted or reduced. Complaints of pain from areas around a joint indicate a possible luxation. Even more important is to ask for symptoms of nerve damage, including permanent or transient numbness and impaired motor function in any part of the arm.

NOTE

It is essential to evaluate nerve function before taking the patient to the operating room.

3.3.2 Clinical Signs and Symptoms

Both the "hard" and the "soft" signs of vascular trauma occur after upper extremity vascular injuries. Examples, in descending frequency of occurrence, include diminished or absent radial pulse, motor deficit, sensory loss, hemorrhage, and expanding hematoma. It is common for a diminished radial pulse or an abnormal brachial blood pressure to be the only sign of vascular obstruction. Because pulse wave propagation through a thrombus is possible, a palpable radial pulse does not completely exclude arterial obstruction; therefore, a high suspicion of arterial injury is necessary even when a palpable pulse is found. As a guideline, a difference of more than 20 mmHg in blood pressure between the arms should make the examiner suspect a vascular injury. Inability to move the fingers, hands, and arms as well as disturbances in sensation are frequently associated with vascular injury. The sensory and motor functions must therefore be carefully examined and evaluated to disclose any nerve damage that should be repaired. A list of what this examination should cover is given in Table 3.2. In unconscious patients, this examination is the only way to reveal indications of arterial damage.

3.4 Diagnostics

Investigations beyond the physical examination of the patient should be done only in stable patients. Accordingly, most patients with distal arm injuries can undergo angiography or duplex scanning provided that these investigations do not delay treatment. Arteriography is indicated when arterial involvement not is obvious. For example, patients with trauma in the elbow region – blunt or penetrating – with clear ischemia and no radial pulse do not need arteriography before surgery.

Table 3.2. Evaluation of nerve function in the arm

Injured nerve (s)	Symptom	Findings
Brachial plexus	Inability to move the arm; limb hangs with extended elbow and forearm pronated	Unable to discriminate sensation on the neck
Axillary nerve	Inability to abduct the arm	Unable to discriminate sensation on the dorsal side of the shoulder
Ulnar nerve	Numbness and inability to move the 5th finger	Unable to discriminate sensation in the pulp of the 5th finger
Median nerve	Inability to flex the hand and numbness in the three middle fingers	Unable to discriminate sensation in the pulp of the index finger
Radial nerve	Numbness and inability to move the thumb	Unable to discriminate sensation in the web between the thumb and index finger

If the patient has multiple injuries, shotgun injuries, or suspected proximal arterial involvement, arteriography is recommended to determine the exact site of injury. Arteriography should also be done when there are indistinct signs of ischemia and arterial injury is only suspected. Included in this indication for arteriography is the so-called proximity injury, referring to injury in patients without signs of distal ischemia but with trauma in close proximity to a major artery. Of patients undergoing arteriography for this indication, 10–20% are reported to have arterial lesions. If the arteriogram reveals injury to the subclavian or axillary artery, endovascular treatment can proceed right away.

Duplex scanning has replaced arteriography in some hospitals and is probably just as accurate in experienced hands. Intimal flaps and small areas of vascular wall thrombosis may be difficult to identify with duplex scanning under some circumstances, but such small lesions in the arm can, on the other hand, usually be treated without exploration.

Computed tomography (CT) angiography is an important modality for diagnosing proximal arterial injuries in particular. It is reported to be at least as accurate as arteriography in this area. The use of CT angiography is likely to increase in the near future because it is quicker than angiography, and most trauma centers have rapid access to good-quality CT.

3.5 Management and Treatment

3.5.1 Management Before Treatment

3.5.1.1 Severely Injured and Unstable Patients

Patients arriving to the emergency department with active serious bleeding after a single injury to an arm are rare. When this does occur, manual direct pressure over the wound can control the bleeding while general resuscitation measures according to Advanced Trauma Life Support principles are undertaken: oxygen, monitoring of vital signs, placement of intravenous (IV) lines, and infusion of fluids (see also Chapter 9, p. 105, for suggestions). It is important not to forget to adminis-

ter analgesics (5–10 mg of an opiate IV) and, when indicated, antibiotics and tetanus prophylaxis.

Multiply injured patients with signs of arm ischemia should be treated according to the hospital's general trauma management protocol, and the vascular injury is usually evaluated during the second survey. Serious ongoing bleeding has high priority, but arm ischemia should be managed after resuscitation and treatment of life-threatening injuries but before orthopedic repair in most circumstances. When the patient has stabilized, arteriography can be performed if indicated (see above).

3.5.1.2 Less Severe Injuries

Most patients with arm injuries arrive in the emergency department in a stable condition without ongoing bleeding but with signs of hand ischemia. For these patients, careful examination of the arm including assessment of nerve function, is essential. Dislocated fractures or luxations should be reduced under proper analgesia. After reduction, examination of vascular function should be repeated. If the radial pulse and distal perfusion return, the position should be stabilized and fixed. Repeated examinations during the following 4 h are mandatory to ensure that the returned perfusion is persistent.

If the vessel injury is definite – an absent radial pulse and reduced hand perfusion – and the site of vascular injury is apparent, the patient can be transferred to the operating room without further diagnostic measures. Patients with findings indicating vascular injury at examination, and those with obvious arterial disruption but with arms so traumatized that the site of arterial injury cannot be determined, should undergo arteriography or duplex scanning. Expediency of repair is required for all locations of arterial injuries in the arm. The proposed time limits indicating a low risk for permanent tissue damage range from 4 h for brachial artery injuries and up to 12 h for forearm injuries. The risk limit for irreversible ischemia following forearm injuries is valid for patients with an incomplete palmar arch. The frequency of this anatomical variation is 20% in most Western populations.

Suspected injuries to the radial and ulnar artery should be treated according to the general principles discussed above. Even cases with nor-

Table 3.3. Allen test

1. Elevate the arm over the head
2. Occlude the radial and ulnar arteries at the wrist
4. Lower the arm
5. Release blood flow through the ulnar artery
6. Inspect and time the return of perfusion
7. Repeat, and release blood flow through the radial artery instead.
8. A return of perfusion >5 s is considered a positive Allen test, and the artery is suspected to be inadequate

mal perfusion in the hand but without a radial pulse should be explored and repaired if reasonably simple. When forearm arterial injury is unclear, the Allen test (Table 3.3) can be added to the examination procedure. A positive Allen test together with a history of trauma to an area in close proximity indicate that the radial or ulnar artery is indeed affected. The wound should then be explored and the traumatized artery inspected and mended. Patients with multiple severe injuries and high-risk patients should not be explored if perfusion to the hand is rendered sufficient. For those circumstances, repeat examinations every hour are mandatory to make sure that perfusion is adequate and stable.

3.5.1.3 Amputation

Some arms with vascular injuries are so extensively damaged that amputation is a treatment option. The decision of when to perform a primary amputation versus trying to repair vessels, nerves, tendons, and muscles is difficult. As a general principle, arms with multiple fractures, nerve disruption, ischemia-time longer than 6 h, and extensive crush injuries involving muscle and skin will never regain function and should be amputated. Another principle is that when four out of the five components of the arm are injured – skin, bone, muscles, and vessels – but there is only minor nerve injury, an attempt to save the arm is reasonable. One must keep in mind, however, that the arm needs at least some protective sensation in order to be functional. Children have a greater chance of regaining a functional arm than adults do, and a generous attitude to surgical repair in children is recommended.

NOTE
The surgeon should not try to save an arm when it only has a small chance of being functional and when repair can be accomplished only at considerable risk.

The mangled extremity severity score (MESS) is a grading system designed to aid the decision process for managing massive upper and lower extremity trauma. A score of 7 or more has been proposed as a cut-off value for indicating when amputation cannot be avoided and should be performed as the primary procedure. In some studies, a score 7 predicted an eventual amputation with 100% accuracy. The basis of the MESS scoring system is given in Table 3.4.

As shown in Table 3.4, a crush injury is regarded as particularly unfavorable. The duration of ischemia is also a significant factor taken into account in the MESS system.

Table 3.4. MESS: Mangled Extremity Severity Score (*BP* blood pressure)

Types	Injury characteristics	Points
Low energy	Stab wounds, simple closed fractures, small-caliber gunshot wounds	1
Medium energy	Open fractures, multiple fractures, dislocations, small crush injuries	2
High energy	Shotgun blasts, high-velocity gunshot wounds	3
Massive crush	Logging, railroad accidents	4
No shock (BP normal)	BP stable at the site and at the hospital	1
Transient hypotension	BP unstable at the site but normalizes after fluid substitution	2
Prolonged hypotension	BP <90 mmHg	3
No distal ischemia	Distal pulses, no signs of ischemia	1
Mild ischemia	Absent or diminished pulses, no signs of ischemia	2[a]
Moderate ischemia	No signals by continuous-wave Doppler, signs of distal ischemia	3[a]
Severe ischemia	No pulse; cool, paralyzed limb; no capillary refill	4[a]
<30 years old patient		1
>30 years old patient		2
>50 years old patient		3

[a] Points are doubled if ischemia lasts longer than 6 h.

3.5.2 Operation

3.5.2.1 Preoperative Preparation

Hemodynamically stable patients are placed on their back with the arm abducted 90° on an arm surgery table. The forearm and hand should be in supination. Peripheral or central IV lines should not be inserted on the injured side. Any continuing bleeding is controlled manually directly over the wound. If the site of injury is the brachial artery or distal to it, a tourniquet can be used to achieve proximal control. It is then placed before draping and should be padded to avoid direct skin contact with the cuff. This minimizes the risk for skin problems during inflation. The arm is washed so the skin over the appropriate artery can be incised without difficulty. The draping should allow palpation of the radial pulse and inspection of finger pulp perfusion. One leg is also prepared in case vein harvest is needed.

The position of the arm is the same for more proximal injuries. Proximal control of high brachial and axillary artery trauma may involve exposure and skin incisions in the vicinity of the clavicle and the neck, so for proximal injuries the draping must also allow incisions at this level.

3.5.2.2 Proximal Control

For distal vessel injury, proximal control can be achieved by inflating the previously placed tourniquet to a pressure around 50 mmHg above systolic pressure. The cuff should be inflated with the arm elevated to minimize bleeding by venous congestion. After inflation, the wound is explored directly at the site of injury.

For more proximal injuries, control is achieved by exposing a normal vessel segment above the wounded area. The most common sites for proximal control in the arm are the axillary artery below the clavicle, and the brachial artery (which is what the artery is called distal to the teres major muscle) somewhere in the upper arm. Some common exposures are described in the Technical Tips box.

3.5.2.3 Exploration and Repair

Distal control is achieved by exploring the wound. Sometimes this requires additional skin incisions. The most common site for vascular damage in the arm is the brachial artery at the elbow level. These injuries occurs, for example, because of supracondylar fractures in children and adults. In such cases, exposure and repair of the brachial artery through an incision in the elbow crease is appropriate. The anatomy is shown in Fig. 3.1, and a brief description of the technique is given in the Technical Tips box. Hematomas should be evacuated to allow inspection of nerves and tendons.

TECHNICAL TIPS
Exposure for Proximal Control of Arteries in the Arm

■ Axillary Artery Below the Clavicle

An 8-cm horizontal incision is made 3 cm below the clavicle (Fig. 3.2). The pectoralis major muscle fibers are split parallel to the skin incision. The pectoralis minor muscle is divided close to its insertion. The nerve crossing the pectoralis minor muscle can also be divided without subsequent morbidity. The axillary artery lies immediately below the fascia together with the vein inferiorly, and the lateral cord of the brachial plexus is located above the artery.

■ Brachial Artery in the Upper Arm

The incision is made along the posterior border of the biceps muscle; a length of 6–8 cm is usually enough (Fig. 3.3). The muscles are retracted medially and laterally, and the artery lies in the neurovascular bundle immediately below the muscles. The sheath is incised and the artery freed from the median nerve and the medial cutaneous nerve that surrounds it.

■ Brachial Artery at the Elbow

The incision is placed 2 cm below the elbow crease and should continue up on the medial side along the artery. If possible, veins transversing the wound should be preserved, but they can be divided if necessary for exposure. The medial insertion of the biceps tendon is divided entirely, and the artery lies immediately beneath it. By following the wound proximally, more of the artery can be exposed (Fig. 3.3). If the origins of the radial and ulnar artery need to be assessed, the wound can be elongated distally on the ulnar side of the volar aspect of the arm. The median nerve lies close to the brachial artery, and it is important to avoid injuring it.

For supracondylar fractures, the brachial artery, the median nerve, and the musculocutaneous nerves must sometimes be pulled out of the fracture site. Before the artery is clamped, the patient is given 50 units of heparin/kg body weight IV. Repair should also be preceded by testing inflow and backflow from the distal vascular bed by temporary tourniquet or clamp release. It is often also wise to pass a #2 Fogarty catheter distally to ensure that no clots have formed. Occasionally, inflow is questionable, and proximal obstruction must be ruled out. This can be done intraoperatively by retrograde arteriography as described in Chapter 4 (p. 44) or by duplex scanning.

As a general principle, all vascular injuries in the arms should be repaired, except when revascularization may jeopardize the patient's life. Arterial ligation should be performed only when amputation is planned. Postoperative arm amputation rates are reported to be 43% if the axillary artery is ligated and 30% at the brachial artery level. Another exception is forearm injuries. When perfusion to the hand is rendered adequate – as assessed by pulse palpation and the Allen test – one of these two arteries can be ligated without

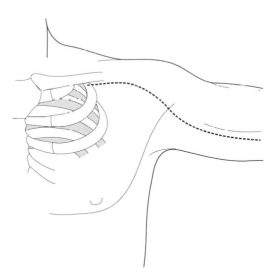

Fig. 3.2. The most proximal part of the axillary artery can be exposed through an incision parallel to and just below the clavicle. Exposure of the brachial artery is through an incision in the medial aspect of the upper arm. This incision can be elongated and connected with the clavicular incision to allow exposure and repair of the entire axillary and brachial artery segments

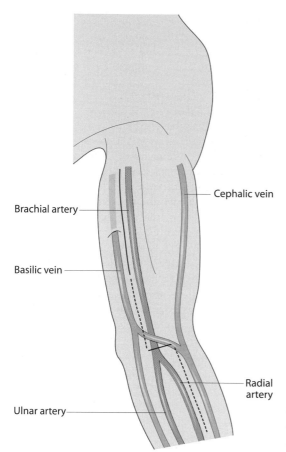

Fig. 3.3. Transverse incision in the elbow for exposing the brachial artery and with possible elongations (*dotted lines*) when access to the ulnar and radial branches as well as to more proximal parts of the brachial artery is needed

morbidity. In a substantial number of patients with differing vessel anatomy, however, ligation of either the ulnar or radial artery may lead to hand amputation. If both arteries are damaged, the ulnar artery should be prioritized because it is usually responsible for the main part of the perfusion to the hand.

For most arterial injuries, vein interposition is necessary for repair. Veins are harvested from the same arm, from parts of the cephalic or basilic vein if the trauma is limited, or from the leg. The saphenous vein in the thigh is suitable for axillary and brachial artery repair, while distal ankle vein pieces can be used for interposition grafts to the

radial and ulnar arteries. Before suturing the anastomoses, all damaged parts of the artery must be excised to reduce the risk of postoperative thrombosis. Rarely, primary suture with and without patching can be used to repair minor lacerations.

Shunting of an arterial injury to permit osteosynthesis is rarely needed in the arm. Vascular interposition grafting can usually be done with an appropriate graft length before final orthopedic repair. Also, extremity shortening due to fractures is less of a problem in the arms (in contrast to the legs), and orthopedic treatment without osteosynthesis is common especially in older patients. Nevertheless, for some arm injuries shunting is a practical technique that allows time for fracture fixation, thus avoiding the risks of redisplacement and repeated vessel injury. One example is injuries to the axillary or brachial artery caused by a proximal humeral fracture, where the fragment needs to be fixed in order to prevent such injuries. Another example is humeral shaft fracture, which needs to be rigidly fixed to abolish the instability that may otherwise endanger the vascular graft. For more details about shunting, see Chapter 9 (p. 111).

Veins should also be repaired if reasonably simple. If the vein injury is caused by a single wound with limited tissue damage, concomitant veins to the distal brachial artery can be ligated. For more extensive injuries where the superficial large veins are likely to be ruined, it is wise to try to repair the deep veins. For very proximal injuries in the shoulder region, vein repair is important to avoid long-term problems with arm swelling. It is also important to cover the mended vessel segment with soft tissue to minimize the risk for infection that may involve the arteries.

3.5.2.4 Finishing the Operation

When the repaired artery or graft's function is doubtful and when the surgeon suspects distal clotting, intraoperative arteriography should be performed. The technique is described in Chapter 10 (p. 128). After completion, all devitalized tissue should be excised and the wound cleaned. For penetrating wounds, damaged tendons and transected nerves should also be sutured. This is not worthwhile for most blunt injuries. Fasciotomy should also be considered before finishing the operation. As in the leg, long ischemia times and successful repair increase the risk of reperfusion and compartment syndrome, but the overall risk for compartment syndrome is reported to be less in the arm than in the leg. For a description of arm fasciotomy techniques, we recommend consulting orthopedic textbooks. After the wounds are dressed, a fractured arm is put into a plaster splint for stabilization.

3.5.2.5 Endovascular Treatment

In contrast to proximal arm vessel trauma, there are few instances in distal injuries when endovascular treatment is a feasible treatment option. Because the brachial artery and the forearm vessels are easy to expose with little morbidity, open repair during exploration of the wound is usually the best option. Possible exceptions to this are treatment of the late consequences of vascular trauma, such as arteriovenous fistulas and pseudoaneurysms.

Especially in the shoulder region, including the axilla, primary endovascular treatment is often the best treatment option. Another circumstance when endovascular treatment is favorable is bleeding from axillary artery branches – such as the circumflex humeral artery – due to penetrating trauma. Active bleeding from branches, but not from the main trunk, observed during arteriography is preferably treated by coiling. The bleeding branches are then selectively cannulated with a guidewire and coiled, using spring coils or injections of thrombin to occlude the bleeding artery.

3.5.3 Management After Treatment

Postoperative monitoring of hand perfusion and radial pulse is recommended at least every 30 min for the first 6 h. When deteriorated function of the repaired artery is suspected, duplex scanning can verify or exclude postoperative problems. Apparent occlusions should be treated by reoperation as soon as possible. Compartment syndrome in the lower arm may also evolve over time, and swelling, muscle tenderness, and rigidity must also be monitored during the initial days. For most patients, treatment with low molecular weight heparin is continued postoperatively. A common dose is 5,000 units subcutaneously twice daily.

Keeping the hand elevated as much as possible may reduce swelling of the hand and arm as well as problems with hematoma formation around the wound. Early mobilization of the fingers facilitate blood flow to the arm and should be encouraged.

3.6 Results and Outcome

The patency of arterial repair in the arm is often excellent, but unfortunately, this appears to have little impact on the eventual arm function. For most patients in whom vessel trauma is associated with nerve and soft tissue injury, it is the nerve function that determines the outcome. Outcome data after arterial repair in upper extremity injuries have been reported in observational studies and case series. One example is a review from the United States of 101 patients with penetrating trauma, including 13 axillary or subclavian cases. Half of the patients had nerve injuries as well. At follow-up the limb salvage rate was 99%, and all patients who needed only vascular repair had excellent functional outcomes. Among arms that required nerve repair, 64% had severe impairment of arm function. The corresponding figure for musculoskeletal repair only was 25%.

A report from the United Kingdom included 28 cases of brachial artery injuries, of which six were blunt. In this study, half of the patients had concomitant nerve injury and underwent immediate nerve repair. All vascular repairs were successful, but the majority of patients undergoing nerve repair appear to have had some functional deficit at follow-up.

Fortunately, it seems that function improves over time in many patients. The risk factors for poor outcome are similar to the ones used for the MESS score – severity of the fracture and soft tissue damage, length of the ischemic period, severity of neurological involvement, and presence of associated injuries.

3.7 Iatrogenic Vascular Injuries

The brachial artery is increasingly being used for cannulation, both for vascular access and for endovascular procedures. The latter requires large introducer sheaths, and it is likely that we will experience an increase in the number of problems related to this. Associated injuries are bleeding and thrombosis. (Both of these issues are discussed in Chapter 12.) Management of bleeding is fairly straightforward. Bleeding is usually easy to control by manual compression; exposure is simple; and repair is often accomplished by a few simple sutures. Thrombosis is much less common but is more complicated to handle. Management should follow the guidelines given in Chapter 4.

Another problem that may be encountered is related to arterial blood sampling from the radial artery. Occasionally, thrombosis of this artery will cause severe arm ischemia. This should then be resolved by embolectomy and patch closure of the injured vessel segment. Sporadically, vein graft interposition is needed. Bleeding or an expanding hematoma due to arterial puncture rarely occurs, but pseudoaneurysm formation is not so infrequent. Such problems should be handled by surgery, including proximal control and patch closure of the injured vessel.

The radial artery is sometimes used as a graft for coronary bypass procedures. This appears to work extremely well, with little late morbidity in the arm where the artery was harvested. We have encountered occasional patients with mild hand ischemia immediately after surgery, but only a few cases who eventually needed revascularization. For these rare patients, a vein bypass from the brachial artery to the site where the ligature was placed at harvest is the recommended treatment.

■ Further Reading

Fields CE, Latifi R, Ivatury RR. Brachial and forearm vessel injuries. Surg Clin North Am 2002; 82(1):105–114

McCready RA. Upper-extremity vascular injuries. Surg Clin North Am 1988; 68(4):725–740

Myers SI, Harward TR, Maher DP, et al. Complex upper extremity vascular trauma in an urban population. J Vasc Surg 1990; 12(3):305–309

Nichols JS, Lillehei KO. Nerve injury associated with acute vascular trauma. Surg Clin North Am 1988; 68(4):837–852

Ohki T, Veith FJ, Kraas C, et al. Endovascular therapy for upper extremity injury. Semin Vasc Surg 1998;11(2):106–115

Pillai L, Luchette FA, Romano KS, et al. Upper-extremity arterial injury. Am Surg 1997; 63(3):224–227

Shaw AD, Milne AA, Christie J, et al. Vascular trauma of the upper limb and associated nerve injuries. Injury 1995; 26(8):515–518

Stein JS, Strauss E. Gunshot wounds to the upper extremity. Evaluation and management of vascular injuries. Orthop Clin North Am 1995; 26(1):29–35

Thompson PN, Chang BB, Shah DM, et al. Outcome following blunt vascular trauma of the upper extremity. Cardiovasc Surg 1993; 1(3):248–250

Acute Upper Extremity Ischemia

4

CONTENTS

■ 4.1 Summary

■ History and physical examination are sufficient for the diagnosis.

■ Few patients need angiography.

■ Embolectomy should be performed in most patients.

■ It is important to search for the embolic source.

■ 4.2 Background and Pathogenesis

Acute ischemia in the upper extremity constitutes 10–15% of all acute extremity ischemia. The etiology is emboli in 90% of the patients. The reason for this higher rate compared with the leg is that atherosclerosis is less common in arm arteries. Emboli have the same origins as in the lower extremity (see Chapter 10, p. 120) and usually end up obstructing the brachial artery. Sometimes plaques or an aneurysm in the subclavian or axillary arteries is the primary source of emboli. Embolization to the right arm is more common than to the left due to the vascular anatomy.

For the 10% of patients with atherosclerosis and acute thrombosis as the main cause for their arm ischemia, the primary lesions are located in the brachiocephalic trunk or in the subclavian artery. Such pathologies are usually asymptomatic due to well-developed collaterals around the shoulder joint until thrombosis occurs, and they cause either micro- or macroembolization.

Other less frequent causes of acute upper extremity ischemia are listed in Table 4.1.

■ 4.3 Clinical Presentation

Acute arm ischemia is usually apparent on the basis of the physical examination. The symptoms are often relatively discreet, especially early after onset. The explanation for this is the well developed collateral system circumventing the brachial artery around the elbow, which is the most common site for embolic obstruction. The "six Ps" – pain, pallor, paresthesia, paralysis, pulselessness,

Table 4.1. Less common causes of acute upper extremity ischemia

Cause	Characteristics
Arteritis	Lesions in distal and proximal arteries
Buerger's disease	Digital ischemia in young heavy smokers
Coagulation disorders	Generalized or distal thrombosis
Raynaud's disease	Digital ischemia

Table 4.2. Frequency of signs and symptoms in patients with acute arm ischemia

Presentation	Percentage
Pulselessness	96
Coldness	94
Pain	85
Paresthesia	45
Dysfunction	45

poikilothermia – are applicable also for acute arm ischemia, but coldness and color changes are more prominent than for the legs. Accordingly, the most common findings in the physical examination are a cold arm with diminished strength and disturbed hand and finger motor functions. Tingling and numbness are also frequent. The radial pulse is usually absent but is pounding in the upper arm proximal to the obstruction.

Gangrene and rest pain appear only when the obstruction is distal to the elbow and affects both of the paired arteries in a finger or in the lower arm. Ischemic signs or symptoms suggesting acute digital artery occlusion in only one or two fingers, imply microembolization.

4.4 Diagnostics

Only the few patients with uncertain diagnosis, and those with a history and physical findings that indicates thrombosis, need additional work-up. Examples include patients with a history of chronic arm ischemia (arm fatigue, muscle atrophy, and microembolization) and bruits over proximal arteries. Angiography should then be performed to reveal the site of the causing lesion. Duplex ultrasound is rarely needed to diagnose acute arm ischemia but may occasionally be helpful.

4.5 Management and Treatment

4.5.1 Management Before Treatment

Even though symptoms and examination findings may be so subtle that conservative treatment is tempting, surgical removal of the obstruction is almost always preferable. It has been suggested that in patients with a lower-arm blood pressure >60 mmHg embolectomy can be omitted, but such a strategy has not to our knowledge been evaluated systematically. In a patient series of nearly symptomless acute arm ischemia, which was left to resolve spontaneously or with anticoagulation as the only treatment, late symptoms developed in up to 45% of the cases. Surgical treatment is also fairly straightforward. It can be performed using local anesthesia and is associated with few complications.

Very often an embolus is a manifestation of severe cardiac disease, so the patient's cardiopulmonary function should be assessed and optimized as soon as possible. Preoperative preparations include an electrocardiogram (ECG) and laboratory tests to guide anticoagulation treatment (see also Chapter 10, p. 25). Heparin treatment is started perioperatively and continued postoperatively in most patients.

NOTE

Embolectomy is the treatment of choice for almost all patients with diagnosis of acute arm ischemia, regardless of the severity of ischemia.

4.5.2 Operation

4.5.2.1 Embolectomy

As mentioned previously, the most common site for embolic obstruction is the brachial artery. Embolectomy of these clots is performed by exposing the brachial artery as described in Chapter 3 (p. 37). The arm is placed on an arm table. We prefer to perform embolectomy using local anesthesia. Often a transverse incision placed over the palpable brachial pulse can be used. If proximal extension of the incision is required, this should be done in parallel with and dorsal to the dorsal aspect of the biceps muscle. It has to be kept in mind that 10–20% of patients may have a different brachial artery anatomy. The most common variation is a high bifurcation of the radial and ulnar arteries, and next in frequency is a doubled brachial artery. The procedure is described in the Technical Tips box.

An alternative location for embolectomy in the arm is to expose the brachial artery in the bicipital groove. A longitudinal incision starting 10 cm above the elbow that is extended proximally is then used.

TECHNICAL TIPS
Embolectomy via the Brachial Artery

Exposure of this vessel is described in Chapter 3. A transverse arteriotomy in the brachial artery is made as close as possible to the bifurcation of the ulnar and radial arteries. The embolectomy is performed in proximal and distal directions with #2 and #3 Fogarty catheters. Separate embolectomy in each branch should be done if technically simple. The Fogarty catheter otherwise slips down into the larger and straighter ulnar artery. The route of the catheter can be checked by palpation at the wrist level when the inflated balloon passes. On the other hand, restored flow in one of the arteries is usually enough for a result that is sufficient for adequate hand perfusion. The arteriotomy is closed with interrupted 6-0 sutures, and distal pulses and the perfusion in the hand are evaluated. If the result is inadequate – poor backflow after embolectomy, absence of pulse, a weak continuous-wave Doppler signal, and questionable hand perfusion – the arteriotomy should be reopened and intraoperative angiography performed (Table 4.3 and Chapter 10, p. 128).

If it is hard to achieve a good inflow, a proximal lesion may cause the embolization or thrombosis. More complicated vascular procedures are then required to reestablish flow. The embolectomy attempt is then discontinued and the patient taken to the angiography suite for a complete examination. If practically feasible, an alternative is to obtain the angiogram in the operating room. Frequently, however, the preferred treatment is endovascular, and this is better done in the angiography suite. Occasionally the films will reveal a proximal obstruction that needs open repair. Examples of such are carotid-subclavian, subclavian-axillary, and axillary-brachial bypasses.

4.5.2.2 Endovascular Treatment

Thrombolysis is as feasible for acute upper extremity ischemia as it is in the leg. The limited ischemia that often occurs after most embolic events because of the collateral network around the elbow also allows the time needed for planning and moving the patient to the angiosuite. The technique involves cannulation in the groin with a 7-French sheath. Long guide wires and catheters are required to reach the occluded site and makes identification of proximal lesions possible. A new arterial puncture in the brachial artery may be necessary for thrombolysis of distal occlusions.

It can be argued that thrombolysis in spite of acceptable results, rarely is needed for treating this disease because open embolectomy can be performed under local anesthesia with good results and little surgical morbidity. The advantages with endovascular treatment are indeed limited. For patients in whom suspicion of thrombosis is strong or when proximal lesions are likely, it should be attempted first. However, case series indicates that results of thrombolysis are inferior for forearm occlusions. In summary, thrombolysis is an alternative but has little to offer in reducing risk or improving outcome compared with embolectomy for most patients.

4.5.3 Management After Treatment

Patients usually regain full function of their hands immediately after the procedure, and postoperative regimens consist of anticoagulation and a search for the embolic source. Heparin or low molecular weight heparin is administered as described in Chapter 10 (p. 129), usually followed by coumadin. The search for cardiac sources may advocate repeated ECGs, echocardiography, and duplex ultrasound of proximal arteries.

4.6 Results and Outcome

The number of salvaged arms after surgical intervention is very high, 90–95%, and arm function is usually fully recovered. The remaining 5–10% represents patients with extensive thrombosis involving many vascular segments and most branches of the distal arteries. The postoperative

Table 4.3. Technique for retrograde intraoperative angiography

1. Control proximal to arteriotomy is achieved by finger compression and/or vessel loop
2. Insert an angiography catheter or a small caliber baby feeding tube through the arteriotomy in retrograde direction
3. Place the tip of the catheter proximal to the suspected obstructing lesion
4. Inject contrast under simultaneous fluoroscopy in lateral projection with a C-arm

mortality is around 10–40% in most patient series, reflecting that embolization often is a consequence of severe cardiac disease. Postoperative mortality is similar for thrombolysis to treat acute arm ischemia, while early technical success is slightly lower or similar. Less favorable results with thrombolysis are achieved when the distal arteries also are obstructed.

■ Further Reading

Baguneid M, Dodd D, Fulford P, et al. Management of acute nontraumatic upper limb ischemia. Angiology 1999; 50(9):715–720

Eyers P, Earnshaw JJ. Acute non-traumatic arm ischaemia. Br J Surg 1998; 85(10):1340–1346

Pentti J, Salenius JP, Kuukasjarvi P, et al. Outcome of surgical treatment in acute upper limb ischaemia. Ann Chir Gynaecol 1995; 84(1):25–28

Ricotta JJ, Scudder PA, McAndrew JA, et al. Management of acute ischemia of the upper extremity. Am J Surg 1983; 145(5):661–666

Whelan TJ Jr. Management of vascular disease of the upper extremity. Surg Clin North Am 1982; 62(3):373–389

Abdominal Vascular Injuries

5

CONTENTS

5.1 Summary

- Up to 25% of patients with abdominal trauma may have major vascular injury.
- Shock out of proportion to the extent of external injury suggests abdominal vascular injury.
- Isolated abdominal injury in patients with shock suggests major vascular injury that requires emergency laparotomy for control.
- After the abdomen is entered, immediate control of the supraceliac aorta should be considered before continuing the operation.
- Retroperitoneal hematomas should not be explored right away unless they are actively bleeding.
- Stopping the procedure after the initial exploration for damage control to allow time for resuscitation in the intensive care unit is often a reasonable initial treatment.
- If the patient's condition allows and if endovascular methods are available, consider placing an aortic balloon from the left brachial artery for temporary occlusion.

■ 5.2 Background

■ 5.2.1 Background

Abdominal vascular trauma is fairly common in modern civilian life and is a highly lethal injury, with overall mortality around 40% in some reported series. The main cause for this high mortality relates to problems transporting injured patients to the hospital fast enough to prevent exsanguination. Furthermore, abdominal vascular injuries are rarely isolated, and other organs are often severely damaged as well. These factors make it essential to resuscitate promptly and establish a rapid diagnosis.

The surgeon managing patients with major abdominal injuries must be experienced with vascular surgical techniques and be able to expose the aorta and its main branches, as well as the vena cava. Dissection and the extensive organ mobilization required for control and repair are often difficult. It is therefore important to develop a routine that can be employed during exploration and control.

■ 5.2.2 Magnitude of the Problem

Major abdominal vascular injury is seen in up to 25% of patients admitted with vascular trauma. Blunt trauma is more common than penetrating trauma in most European countries, while the opposite is reported in areas where gunshot wounds are more frequent. Abdominal injury represents 10–20% of all traumas to the body caused by road traffic accidents. Major vascular injury is estimated to occur in about 10% of cases of penetrating stab wounds in the abdomen and in about 25% of gunshot wounds. Blunt abdominal trauma affects major vessels less frequently, estimates of below 5% is common in the literature.

NOTE

Major vascular injury is rather common after abdominal trauma.

■ 5.2.3 Etiology and Pathophysiology

■ 5.2.3.1 Penetrating Injury

Penetrating injury creates the types of damage that are common for most arteries – transection, laceration, intimal dissection, and thrombosis, as well as false aneurysms and arteriovenous fistula formation. The first two are more common after stab wounds. Gunshot wounds inflict more widespread damage to the vessel wall, depending on the bullet's velocity. For example, high-velocity missiles at speeds >700 m/sec cause up to 20 times more damage than low-velocity projectiles. An artery located within 10–15 cm of the trajectory regularly thromboses after a high-velocity gunshot injury.

■ 5.2.3.2 Blunt Injury

Typically, blunt injury to abdominal vessels occurs after road traffic accidents or falls from heights. Most commonly damaged are upper abdominal arteries and veins such as the infrarenal aorta. The mechanism is compression of the aorta against the lumbar spine by the steering wheel, especially when seat belts are not used. This causes intimal tears and thrombosis of the aorta. Full-blown rupture has also been reported. Vessel injuries are much less frequent when seat belts are used. Avulsion of branches is also common and there is a high incidence of associated injury to the small arteries. Veins are usually not affected by blunt trauma, except for the left renal vein. Major abdominal injuries may cause avulsion of arteries; in descending order of occurrence the vessels injured are the left renal vein, the renal arteries, the superior mesenteric artery (SMA), and the abdominal aorta just distal to the renal arteries.

■ 5.2.3.3 Pathophysiology

When an artery is perforated, blood extravasates into surrounding tissues, causing a hematoma that counteracts the blood pressure and facilitates spontaneous closure of the hole in the vessel. When a vein is damaged, tamponade of the bleeding often occurs, especially if retroperitoneal, unless the peritoneum is torn or is entered during laparotomy. If vein damage is caused by a pelvic fracture a cavity is created around the fragments, preventing effective tamponade, and the bleeding continues. Venous and arterial bleeding within the mesentery is also enhanced by the same mechanism. The high blood flow through major arteries in the abdomen makes spontaneous cessation of bleeding less likely. Even the aorta, however, has been reported to seal spontaneously after penetrating trauma when it is completely transected. If an artery is partially lacerated, the severed ends cannot contract; the hole is held open, and blood flows more easily into the abdominal cavity. Patients rarely survive for long in this circumstance.

There are two principle mechanisms of vascular injury in blunt abdominal trauma: compression and deceleration forces. The former may cause crush injuries and intramural hematoma or lacerations. The latter cause stretching that creates tension between fixed and movable organs, leading to avulsion or intimal disruption and thrombosis.

5.2.3.4 Associated Injuries

Any and all organs within the abdomen may be injured in association with a major vessel injury. A general rule is that for every major vascular injury, three to four other organs are damaged as well. The rate depends on the etiology of the trauma, the location on the abdominal wall where the impact or wound is located, and the direction of the traumatic force. Table 5.1 gives an estimation of the likelihood of injury to individual organs in association with major vascular injury.

In general, blunt injury is more commonly associated with injury to many other organs, while this is slightly less likely for penetrating trauma. The small bowel is often injured by blunt trauma, and the kidneys and spleen are frequently damaged in both trauma types.

5.3 Clinical Presentation

5.3.1 Medical History

In patients who arrive to the emergency department in shock with signs of penetrating or blunt abdominal injury, the medical history does not add much to the management, although information about the mechanism of trauma is useful when estimating the risk of associated injuries (Table 5.1). Knowing exactly when the injury occurred and when the patient became unconscious may assist in predicting outcome.

Stable patients allows more time to gather information, and it is possible to ask direct questions about the injury. This may provide important clues about the possibility for major vascular injury. For example, patients with contained hematomas are either stable or have a history of a transient hypotensive period. This information is easy to get from Emergency medical personnel. Patients complaining of increasing abdominal pain after either penetrating or blunt trauma should be suspected of bleeding intraabdominally, especially if the blood pressure is decreasing. Shoulder pain and pain when breathing indicate referred pain from blood irritating the diaphragm. Patients should be asked about leg pain as an indication of arterial occlusion or embolization; this is particularly important after blunt trauma. A history of hematuria indicates renal or bladder trauma.

Table 5.1. Probability of organ injury together with major arterial injury in the abdomen (compiled from seven case series)

	Stabbing	Gunshot	Blunt trauma
Liver	+	++	+++
Pancreas	++	+	++
Stomach	+	++	++
Kidney	+++	++	++
Spleen	++	+	+++
Duodenum	+	+	–
Small bowel	+	++	++
Colon	++	++	+

5.3.2 Clinical Signs and Symptoms

The patient who presents with shock a short time after injury to the abdomen should be presumed to have a major vascular injury, with bleeding directly into the peritoneal cavity. Increasing abdominal distension or persistent hypotension despite aggressive resuscitation are other signs suggestive of continuing bleeding from an injured vessel, liver, or spleen. Shock out of proportion to the extent of external injuries, including fractures, suggests abdominal vascular injury as the cause of the bleeding. The finding of a mass during palpation, which is sometimes enlarging and pulsating, strongly suggests major vessel damage. The anatomical location gives some hint about the specific vessel injured.

NOTE

Abdominal distension and shock out of proportion to the extent of external injuries indicate major vascular trauma.

In stable patients, assessment should include the location of the wounds to assess the likelihood for intraabdominal injury. As a general rule, all penetrating wounds between the nipple line and the groin should be presumed to have penetrated the abdominal wall. Penetrating wounds in the midline carry a substantial risk for aortic and vena caval injury, but lateral wounds can also cause injury to these structures. Wounds around the umbilicus indicates that the bifurcation of these vessels is likely to be affected. Entrance wounds located below the umbilicus suggest iliac vessel injury. A trajectory of a gunshot wound that passes the midline also indicated major vascular trauma. It has to be remembered, however, that it is notoriously difficult to assess trajectories, and bone and even the muscle fascia may deflect bullets. The victim's body position at the time of injury can also influence which structures are damaged. Intraabdominal injuries may also be a result of wounds to the back and buttocks.

Large hematomas tend to cause abdominal distension and tenderness in conscious patients. Tenderness may also be a result of peritonitis due to contamination by perforated bowel or bowel ischemia. Blood in the urine, rectum, vagina, or a nasogastric tube also indicates intraperitoneal penetration. Signs of a pelvic fracture should lead to a high suspicion for iliac vessel damage.

Distal ischemia should also be excluded, and palpation of pulses in the groins and distally is obligatory after any major trauma. Particularly after blunt trauma, distal ischemia may be the only sign suggesting vessel damage. Unfortunately, 25% of patients who experience blunt trauma causing some degree of arterial obstruction have normal femoral pulses. Physical examination should also include an assessment of the "six Ps" (see Chapter 10, p. 121). In hemodynamically stable patients with abnormal pulse examination, the ankle–brachial index (ABI) should be measured to aid in assessing limb ischemia. An ABI <0.9 – especially unilaterally – implies some degree of vessel obstruction. In general, trauma patients tend to be young and therefore do not have significant atherosclerosis, so an asymmetrical ABI could be the only clue to an occult vascular injury. Penetrating injury together with absent pulses strongly indicates trauma to a major axial artery.

5.4 Diagnostics

In some circumstances, patients are so unstable that they must be taken to the operating room for laparotomy without diagnostic procedures. In stable multitrauma patients in whom laparotomy is not indicated for other reasons, additional diagnostic measures may identify major vascular injury, determine the extent of damage to other organs, and facilitate treatment planning.

Ultrasonography can and should be performed in most patients with abdominal trauma, regardless of their condition. The abdomen can be scanned in the emergency department without moving the patient and often takes less than 10 min to perform. Its main objective is to detect hemoperitoneum as a possible source of hypotension. It may also detect large hematomas and pseudoaneurysms, but often misses retroperitoneal hemorrhage. Ultrasound also has low sensitivity for detecting and excluding injuries to other organs such as the intestines, liver, spleen, and kidneys.

Computed tomography (CT) has become a valuable and widely used tool for evaluating most stable patients with abdominal trauma. The CT scan provides detailed information about the ret-

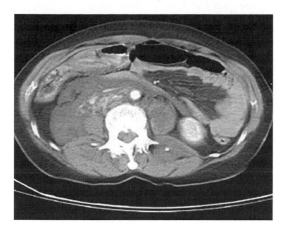

Fig. 5.1. An example of computed tomography showing retroperitoneal bleeding caused by blunt abdominal trauma

roperitoneal space, presence of hemoperitoneum, active bleeding, false aneurysms, and damage to other organs. The main limitation is its inability to identify intestinal perforation, diaphragmatic injuries, and mesenteric tears. For blunt trauma it gives information about the extent of damage to the liver and spleen and thereby often identifies patients who do not need laparotomy and those who should undergo arteriography. Because CT is unreliable in diagnosing intestinal perforation, it has not been as valuable after penetrating trauma. The use of contemporary spiral CT with intravenous contrast has made it possible to detect active bleeding, missile paths, and visceral perforation in both blunt and penetrating trauma. For most abdominal vascular injuries in stable patients, it is an excellent screening tool, and when enhanced by contrast, bleeding and vessel thrombosis can also be diagnosed. Examples include detection of renal and visceral artery injuries, as seen in Fig. 5.1.

Some authors have recently suggested that CT should be performed even in unstable patients in order to reduce the number of unnecessary laparotomies. This concept depends in part on the availability of CT, its location in the hospital and on a strict management protocol.

Angiography is rarely used today to diagnose arterial injury after abdominal trauma. Exceptions are stable patients with no signs of peritonitis for whom a CT scan has given some indirect evi-

dence of arterial damage. The arteriogram is then the initial step in an endovascular procedure for definite treatment. Examples are arteriovenous fistulas, pseudoaneurysm, active bleeding from branch vessels, liver and spleen injuries, and pelvic fractures. Other indications for angiography are to diagnose suspected minor arterial lesions after blunt trauma and to assess patients with signs of organ or distal ischemia. Examples include aortic and renal artery intimal tears and thrombosis.

A plain x-ray may be indicated in patients with gunshot wounds in order to locate the bullet, to facilitate estimation of the trajectory after applying markers at the entry and exit sites. If the bullet is suspected to have passed through regions where major vessels are located, angiography may be indicated. Plain x-ray can also identify gas in the abdominal cavity. Most of this information can also be gained from CT.

Diagnostic peritoneal lavage (DPL) was the standard way to diagnose intraabdominal bleeding before the CT era. Because of its invasiveness and the very high sensitivity in detecting even minute intraabdominal bleedings that often does not need surgical repair, it is much less often performed today. Furthermore, it may not detect even significant retroperitoneal bleeding. DPL is indicated in unstable patients when it is vital to determine the source of bleeding and when ultrasound is inconclusive and CT not possible to perform. It may also be considered in stable patients when CT and ultrasound are not available or in multitrauma patients who require neurological or orthopedic operations and therefore will be inaccessible for evaluation for long time periods. Technical details about DPL are beyond the scope of this text, so for descriptions on how to carry out DPL, we recommend textbooks on abdominal trauma.

Intravenous pyelography (IVP) is a tool for diagnosing renal vascular injury that largely has been replaced by CT. It may still have a place in the operating room because it can be used during surgery. The sign of renal vascular injury is lack of the appearance of contrast in one of the kidneys. Its main limitation is low sensitivity, and up to a third of patients with vascular injury have normal IVPs

Laparoscopy has yet to find its place for evaluating patients with suspected abdominal vascular injury. It requires an operating suite and general anesthesia, it cannot easily evaluate the retroperitoneal space, and even small amounts of intraabdominal bleeding may disturb visualization. Its main advantage is reported to be diagnosis of diaphragmatic injuries in stable patients.

5.5 Management and Treatment

5.5.1 Management Before Treatment

5.5.1.1 Treatment and Management in the Emergency Department

The early management should follow the ABCs of trauma resuscitation. Patients in shock should be intubated and ventilated with 100% oxygen, and at least two large intravenous (IV) lines should be inserted, preferably in the upper extremity. Fluid replacement through vascular access in the lower extremities may extravasate and not reach the heart if pelvic veins or the vena cava are injured. The strategy and technique for obtaining rapid venous access in trauma are described in Chapter 11, p. 137. When the lines are in place blood should be drawn for routine analysis and blood typing and cross-matching. Laboratory studies follow standard trauma management and should also include acid-base balance, serum amylase, and urineanalysis. Fluid resuscitation with warm lactated Ringer's solution is continued or started. If the patient has obvious severe blood loss, blood and plasma are added as soon as possible. Platelet substitution should also be considered. A Foley catheter and a nasogastric tube should be inserted in all patients with abdominal trauma. Hypothermia must be prevented by all means.

Physical examination should be done during the second survey, and the findings lead the management. For some patients, further diagnostic procedures will determine whether they require surgery or nonsurgical treatment. Ultrasound, for instance, performed in the emergency department can rule out or verify intraabdominal bleeding. Patients with associated thoracic injury should undergo chest x-ray to detect hemothorax and other thoracic injuries as possible sources of bleeding. However, as outlined below, CT is now the most important diagnostic modality for stable patients.

5.5.1.2 Unstable Patients

The management of unstable patients is summarized in Table 5.2. Patients in shock with isolated abdominal injury should undergo emergency laparotomy. An abdominal ultrasound scan is needed in multiply injured patients with injuries in the thorax, head, or extremities. Unstable patients with multiple injuries and a negative ultrasound scan are a specific diagnostic problem. It may be worthwhile to pursue the evaluation to rule out abdominal bleeding as a possible cause of hypotension in these patients. If they are in severe shock, DPL may be indicated to rule out intraabdominal origin of the bleeding. CT may also be an option in "less" unstable patients, especially if there is improvement with resuscitation and CT is readily available.

NOTE

Unstable patients with a negative ultrasound scan pose a particular diagnostic problem when trying to exclude a major vascular abdominal injury.

If DPL is negative, the cause of bleeding is likely to be outside the abdomen, but false negatives can occur. DPL may miss a serious retroperitoneal bleeding. The ultimate management will then be a matter of clinical judgment regarding whether the patient will tolerate a CT scan or must be moved to the operating room for emergency laparotomy. The boxes in Table 5.2 indicating "maybe" represent circumstances in which clinical judgment is especially important for the management.

If the patient is severely unstable and probably not tolerates examination with CT, DPL could possibly rule out intraperitoneal hemorrhage. A positive DPL is an indication for surgery, while a negative DPL points to the need for continued evaluation as discussed above. More resuscitation, for example, may be attempted followed by a CT scan under close surveillance.

Emergency Thoracotomy

Patients with penetrating abdominal injury who are unconscious and have prolonged severe hypotension (<70 mmHg) but no other apparent injuries causing the shock may occasionally be saved by immediate proximal control of the aorta in the emergency/operating room. Cross-clamping

Table 5.2. Management of abdominal injuries when vascular damage is suspected

Patient's condition	Other injuries	Ultrasonography		Computed tomography		Diagnostic peritoneal lavage		Surgery
			Finding		Finding		Finding	
Unstable	No	No (Yes[a])		No		No		Yes
	Yes	Yes	Positive	No		No		Yes
			Negative	Maybe		Maybe	Positive	Yes
							Negative	Maybe
Stable	Yes/no	No		Yes	Positive	No		Maybe
					Negative	No		Observation

[a]After blunt trauma, all patients should undergo ultrasonography.

of the descending thoracic aorta through a thoracotomy in the 4th or 5th interspace may then be attempted if the patient is believed to have a realistic chance of survival (e.g., became moribund in the emergency department or lost measurable blood pressure during the last part of the transport to the hospital). The technique is briefly summarized in Chapter 2 (p. 22). Aortic clamping before laparotomy can facilitate perfusion through the coronary and carotid arteries and prevent further bleeding during laparotomy. Deterioration is common in these severely ill patients when the abdominal wall is incised and the tamponade it maintains is released. It is disappointing, however, how seldom this maneuver leads to the patient's survival.

5.5.1.3 Stable Patients

Stable patients with clinical signs of peritonitis after penetrating trauma should undergo laparotomy without delay for diagnostic procedures. All others – with either blunt or penetrating trauma – should be evaluated with CT to reveal the extent of injury (Table 5.2). If ultrasonography in the emergency department is performed routinely in all trauma patients, it can be added to the diagnostic process, but most stable patients admitted after blunt trauma will need CT scanning regardless of ultrasound findings. For example, surgery is indicated for patients with ongoing active bleeding, aortic thrombosis, or large hematomas caused by organ injury. For other injuries, such as branch vessel bleeding, renal or SMA thrombosis, and pelvic arterial injuries, angiography followed by endovascular treatment is often the best option.

Stable patients undergoing CT must be supervised at all times because they may become unstable quickly. Personnel must therefore be skilled in assessing vital signs and the abdomen throughout the examination.

5.5.1.4 Laparotomy or Not?

Unnecessary laparotomy is performed in up to 25% of patients with abdominal trauma and is associated with considerable morbidity and cost. Nonoperative treatment has therefore grown in popularity but has to be balanced against the price of missed injuries. This approach has increased the need for additional diagnostic procedures to aid the decision process. Table 5.2 summarizes these diagnostic modalities and how they can be used for managing the patients.

Nonoperative treatment is particularly appealing in stable and multitrauma patients. Examples of injuries that may be treated nonoperatively are some liver, spleen, and renal injuries. For detailed discussion on this subject, we recommend textbooks on trauma. Vascular injuries may be treated without open surgery using endovascular methods. One example is embolization of bleeding pelvic vessels caused by pelvic fractures; another is renal artery injuries.

5.5.1.5 Renal Artery Injuries

The most common type of renal vascular injury after blunt trauma is thrombosis. This is usually diagnosed by CT. For most blunt injuries, nonoperative treatment is appropriate if there are no other indications for operative intervention, such as when the diagnosis is made more than 12 h after the trauma occurred. Reconstruction attempts after renal ischemia of over 10–12 h are usually futile, and the kidney will not regain its function if this time limit is passed; however, successful revascularization has been performed after 24 h of ischemia. Exceptions when salvage may be tried after longer ischemia times, are bilateral renal ischemia, and patients with retrograde blood flow as observed on an arteriogram indicating some collateral supply.

Renal artery thrombosis following trauma can usually be treated by angioplasty and stenting, provided that rapid access to the angiosuite is possible. Also, minor lesions such as intimal flaps in the renal arteries do not always need surgical treatment. Such minor lesions should be treated by observation. This includes patients with segmental parenchymal ischemia. Accordingly, surgical reconstruction is saved for patients with active bleeding and for situations when the diagnosis is made during laparotomy.

5.5.2 Operation

5.5.2.1 Preoperative Preparation

The following section describes the recommended procedure for a patient with active intraabdominal bleeding. It is also applicable for stable patients in whom more time is initially available. Regardless, the patient should be prepped from the chin to the knees so thoracic and groin vessel access is possible if required. The saphenous vein must also be accessible for harvest. After the patient is prepped and draped and the surgeon is dressed and ready, the patient is quickly anesthetized followed by the start of the operation.

5.5.2.2 Exploration

Exploration

A midline incision from the xiphoid process to the pubic bone is best for most situations. It is important to divide fat and fascia for the entire length of the wound before the peritoneum is incised. The peritoneum is then opened rapidly – particularly if the blood pressure drops after the abdomen is entered – and the lesser omentum is opened and widened using fingers. The aorta is palpated with the index finger and can be occluded manually or by compressing it against the spine with an aortic occluder. To perform this maneuver it is sometimes necessary to mobilize the left lobe of the liver to the right, as described in Chapter 7 (pp. 83, 84). If the hematoma is located above the transverse mesocolon and aortic compression does not rise the blood pressure, supraceliac or juxtaceliac bleeding should be suspected. Extension of the incision into the thoracic area to obtain occlusion of the descending thoracic aorta is then recommended. This can be accomplished by dividing the diaphragmatic crura and rarely requires median sternotomy.

The aortic compression or occlusion is maintained while evacuating blood and blood clots. Remember that blood clots tend to accumulate close to the bleeding site. Next, all sites where active bleeding is noticed or suspected are packed with laparotomy pads. Such pads usually stop even quite substantial bleeding from the liver and spleen as well as all venous bleedings, including bleeding from the vena cava. Bleeding from the aorta, iliac, celiac axis, SMA, and renal arteries, on the other hand, will usually continue despite packing if the aortic occlusion is released and the patient not is hypotensive. Visual large arterial hemorrage may be handled without further dissection, by ligature but one must be careful not to interrupt the proximal SMA, aorta, or the renal arteries. Temporary shunting may be a solution for these vessels.

So far the whole procedure should take less than 10–20 min.

NOTE

For patients in shock, the peritoneum is left intact until the fascia is opened in its entire length to preserve the peritoneal tamponade as long as possible.

At this point, bleeding sources and their seriousness are assessed. If the patient is hypothermic and has coagulopathy, the best decision could be to stop the procedure, to temporarily close the abdomen and continue resuscitation in the intensive care unit. This option, or "damage control" break, may be considered even with some continuing active bleeding. Damaged bowel segments are ligated and injured ureters externalized before temporary closure of the skin. The other option is to continue the operation by focusing on definite control of the most severe bleeding sites.

NOTE

Aortic compression at the supraceliac level is often a good way to achieve temporary proximal control while assessing the damage.

Exposure and Control

Before the operation for definitive control continues, packing is reinforced by adding more pads. Those packs should reapproximate disrupted tissue planes if possible. Minor bleeding sites should be left for later, unless they disturb the surgical field. If the main bleeding appears to come from the aorta at the suprarenal or juxtarenal level, the manual supraceliac aortic occlusion is changed to a clamp. During the time needed for the initial exploration described before, resuscitation can often improve the patient's condition enough to allow temporary release of the aortic occlusion. If not, it is often wise to wait a while before trying to clamp the supraceliac aorta more permanently. The aorta is freed by finger dissection, sporadically aided by cutting the muscle fibers from the diaphragmatic crus with a long-bladed pair of scissors. This exposure is necessary for clamp placement. The

technique is further described in Chapter 7 (p. 84). While the exposure also gives satisfactory proximal control to repair infrarenal aortic injuries, the clamp should be moved to an infrarenal site as soon as possible. If the patient's condition allows and endovascular methods are available, the placement of an aortic balloon through a left brachial or femoral artery access, is of great potential value. This is best performed in the operating room. It makes temporary occlusion of the aorta at different levels possible in case of uncontrollable bleeding during dissection. The technique is also described in Chapter 7 (p. 83).

The technique for vascular exposure and final control of other bleeding sites is described in the Technical Tips box. Active bleeding from arteries and veins around the liver hilus can be controlled by using the "Pringle maneuver" – digital occlusion of the hepatoduodenal ligament – followed by careful dissection of the separate vessels.

NOTE

Stopping the procedure after the initial exploration of damage control to allow time for resuscitation in the intensive care unit is often a reasonable initial treatment.

TECHNICAL TIPS
Exposure of Different Intraabdominal Vascular Segments

■ Suprarenal Aorta and its Branches

The best way to expose the suprarenal aorta, the origin of the SMA, the celiac axis, and the left renal artery is to perform a "left medial visceral rotation." Divide the peritoneal reflection of the descending colon, release the splenic flexure, and cut the attachments between the spleen and the diaphragm. Rotate the table slightly to the right and move all viscera, including the colon, small bowel, spleen, and the gastric fundus, to the right side of the abdomen and cover all organs in large, moist lap pads. This maneuver can be employed either in a plane dorsal to the left kidney – which will include the kidney with the viscera rotated to the right – or ventral to the kidney. It is slightly more difficult to find the appropriate dissection plane for the latter approach, but this is more

practical for repairing most injuries. On the other hand, including the left kidney with the rotated viscera gives access to the posterior wall of the aorta. When performed, little additional dissection enables proximal control using a Satinsky clamp. The clamp is placed as distal as possible on the aorta but sufficiently above the wounded area to permit repair. Distal control is achieved by clamps, balloons, or a Foley catheter.

Injuries to the portal vein are exposed and controlled by dividing the head of the pancreas between clamps or staplers to control the superior mesenteric and splenic veins. Sometimes the gastroduodenal artery must be divided to facilitate exposure. (See Fig. 5.2.)

▼

TECHNICAL TIPS
Exposure of Different Intraabdominal Vascular Segments (*continued*)

■ Vena Cava and Right Renal Vein and Artery

Exposure of the infrahepatic vena cava and the right side of aorta, including the portal vein and the distal part of the SMA, is initiated by dividing the attachments of the ascending colon, including the hepatic flexure. Mobilize the colon, duodenum, and the head of pancreas medially – perform a full "Kocher maneuver" by dividing the lateral, superior, and inferior attachments of the duodenum – and cover the organs in lap pads and place them under retractors. When the dissection is continued through the hematoma, the renal vein is encountered first. To enable mobilization upward and downward, it is banded and freed from surrounding tissue. The renal artery is usually located below or somewhat cranially to the vein. Proximal control of the renal artery is accomplished either on the left side of the vena cava or below the renal vein. A DeBakey clamp is used unless the injury is located close to the arterial origin; then partial aortic occlusion with a larger clamp is necessary. As shown in Fig. 5.2, venous control is accomplished by digital or sponge-stick compression of the vena cava distal and proximal to the wounded area. Another option for control during vena cava repair is to insert a Foley catheter into the injured vessel and inflate the balloon in the hole. Dorsal cava injuries at the level of the renal vein sometimes necessitate mobilization and medial rotation of the right kidney to expose the wounded area. This approach is also the best way to expose the portal vein within the head of the pancreas. The reason why it works is that it is the most dorsal structure in the portal triad (Fig. 5.3).

■ Retrohepatic Vena Cava

First, the inflow to the liver – the hepatic artery and portal vein – is clamped together with the bile duct. Use a small angled vascular clamp. Second, the infrahepatic vena cava is freed as described above and carefully cross-clamped proximal to the renal veins. Third, the proximal aorta is exposed to be ready for cross-clamping if the patient becomes hypotensive due to the cava disruption. This exploration is performed through

the omentum minus as described in the main text. The recommendation is to clamp the aorta if the blood pressure falls to 60 mmHg or less. If possible, infrarenal cross-clamping is employed, especially if clamping is required for a long time to achieve vascular repair. The fourth step is to mobilize the liver by dividing all hepatic ligaments – the falciform, teres, and right and left triangular ligaments – and clamp the suprarenal cava. This must be done with care so the bleeding does not increase. Control of the proximal vena cava can be achieved below the diaphragm by continuing the blunt and sharp dissection through the falciform ligament. At this level the vena cava is freed circumferentially to permit clamping well above the hepatic veins. Sometimes supradiaphragmatic exposure is necessary. A right anterolateral incision is then made in the diaphragm, and the dissection is continued by opening the dorsal pericardial fold until the suprahepatic vena cava is reached. Finally, the liver is mobilized upward from the right and left to expose as much as possible of the retrohepatic vena cava.

■ Infrarenal Aorta

The aorta is exposed as for elective aortic procedures. Wrap the small bowel in moist lap pads and move it to the right side of the abdomen. Incise the peritoneal reflection over the distal portions of the duodenum and mobilize it to the right and cephalad. Open the peritoneum directly over the infrarenal aorta and free it from surrounding tissue so that a clamp can be placed proximal to the injury. Another clamp distally or a Foley catheter inserted in the hole is used for distal control. If the injury is in one of the common iliac arteries or is close to the bifurcation, the iliac arteries must be controlled distally. Dissection and clamping of particularly the right common iliac artery must be done with care so the iliac vein located underneath not is damaged. If the iliac veins are injured, exposure sometimes necessitates temporary division of the iliac artery to reach the injured vein. Control is obtained by manual compression.

▼

■ Iliac Arteries and Veins

The iliac arteries on the right side are found after mobilizing the small bowel to the left and the cecum proximally. The left-sided arteries are found after mobilizing the sigmoid colon to the right and incising the peritoneum. The arteries and veins are usually quite easy to separate and control at this level.

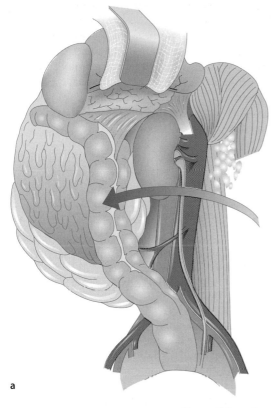

a

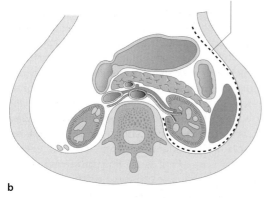

Plane of Dissection

b

Fig. 5.2. Medial rightward rotation of the left viscera, exposing the aorta from the diaphragm and all the way down to the iliac arteries ("left medial visceral rotation")

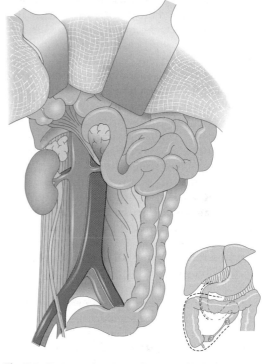

Fig. 5.3. Peritoneal incision for a "Kocher maneuver" to mobilize the duodenum, small intestine, and right colon for a "right medial visceral rotation." This allows exposure of the entire inferior vena cava, right renal, and iliac vessels

It is necessary to have previous experience in liver surgery to successfully accomplish "total" control of liver injuries, and the medial visceral rotation for suprarenal aortic and cava exposure may also be very difficult without experience.

Retrohepatic Injuries. Particularly cumbersome is control of injuries to the retrohepatic vena cava. This type of exposure is difficult because the liver covers the entire anterior surface of the vena cava. The low number of patients surviving long enough to arrive at the hospital with this type of injury also makes it hard for most surgeons to gather experience with it. The special problems encountered concern the difficult access (because, as stated, the liver covers the vena cava) and the reduced blood volume returning to the heart when the vena cava is clamped.

A number of methods have been suggested for control. One example is atriocaval shunting by inserting a large tube into the vena cava through a hole in right atrium's appendage. In the Technical Tips box, the technique for total clamping and control directly without adjunctive measures is described because we feel this may occasionally be a practical approach for controlling unmanageable bleeding from this area. For immediate control during the exploratory procedure for total control (clamping the aorta, the infrarenal vena cava, and the suprahepatic vena cava and doing the Pringle maneuver), the liver is compressed dorsally against the spine manually and by using lap pads. Control of bleeding by direct pressure is facilitated by dividing the falciform ligament and tilting the liver downward. However, it is reasonable to refrain from attempting to repair injuries to the retrohepatic vena cava and instead, as the only measure taken, pack the liver to reduce the bleeding.

> **NOTE**
>
> It is rarely sensible to try to repair retrohepatic vena cava injuries in unstable patients.

Superior Mesenteric Artery Injuries. SMA injuries can also be quite difficult to expose and control. The importance of the SMA for perfusing the intestine makes SMA injuries particularly cumbersome to manage. Delaying restoration of flow more than 4–6 h inevitably leads to bowel necrosis and possibly death. "Medial visceral rotation" or "high" infrarenal aortic exposure provides access to the first 3–4 cm of the SMA, but the next part of the vessel is incorporated in the pancreas. Surgical hematomas in this area make the dissection even more difficult. Therefore, it has been suggested that the pancreas shall be divided to expose SMA injuries. Another option is to leave the injured area and perform a bypass from the aorta to a distal part of the SMA and ligate it at its origin. When a large hematoma around the head of the pancreas is encountered and the bowel is ischemic, the middle part of the SMA is probably injured, and such a bypass can be attempted for maintaining bowel perfusion.

> **NOTE**
>
> The aorta, the renal arteries, and the proximal part of the SMA should not be ligated for control during damage control surgery.

▍ *Retroperitoneal Hematomas*

Particularly after blunt trauma, intact retroperitoneal hematomas are a common finding during laparotomy. If such hematomas are not bleeding actively or expanding, they should not be explored right away. Other injuries can be treated first if needed and if sufficient time is available, additional diagnostic work-up pursued. Hematomas with signs of active bleeding and those that appear to be expanding rapidly should be left intact until proximal and distal control is achieved.

Even small hematomas can harbor significant vessel injuries.

When the surgeon is selecting the approach for vascular exposure and control, the location of the hematoma should be considered. A midline hematoma superior to the transverse mesocolon indicates injury to the suprarenal aorta or its branches. If combined with ischemic bowel signs, injury to the SMA should be suspected. Blood in the area of the portal triad suggests hepatic artery or portal vein injury. A midline infrarenal aortic or vena cava injury is suspected when the hematoma is located below the mesocolon. Lateral peritoneal hematomas occur after renal vessel and parenchymal injuries. A pelvic hematoma indicate iliac vessel damage.

Because of their propensity to contain major vessel damage, it is recommended to explore most hematomas in the midline. As mentioned in the section on management (page 51), contained kidney and renal vessel injuries after blunt trauma can often be treated nonsurgically. Therefore, lateral hematomas found after blunt injury should be left intact. A common opinion is that, after penetrating injury, lateral hematomas should be explored because they are more often associated with major vessel damage. Our recommendation, however, is to leave all nonexpanding lateral hematomas, regardless of trauma mechanism. Instead, the patient should undergo CT, IVP, or angiography to rule out major vessel injury and urinary leaks.

The most common cause of pelvic hematomas after blunt trauma is pelvic fracture. Hematomas in this area should not be explored routinely. Even if the pelvic hematoma is expanding, it is often better to pack the pelvic area and continue the work-up with arteriography. For penetrating trauma, on the other hand, it is usually wise to explore pelvic hematomas after securing proximal control to exclude vessel damage.

5.5.2.4 Vessel Repair

The principles of repair are similar to those for all other vascular injuries in the body. Lacerations can be sutured directly, using polypropylene suture appropriate to the vessel size. For larger holes a patch is used to avoid vessel narrowing. Vein is the preferred material. Complete transections can occasionally be sutured end to end, but interposition grafting by using a saphenous vein is usually needed. For renal, SMA, and celiac axis arterial repair, the saphenous vein can be used as it is, but for aortic injuries larger sizes are required. Then, and if the abdomen is contaminated by perforated bowel, a vein graft – which is more infection resistant – is manufactured by suturing several vein pieces together as described on Chapter 15, p. 189. Otherwise, expanded polytetrafluoroethylene (ePTFE) or polyester grafts can be used. Severely damaged vessels must be debrided to provide intact vessel walls before the anastomoses are sutured. Vein lacerations and transection are treated in exactly the same way as arteries. Some vessels in the abdomen can also be ligated without significant morbidity. This is discussed below, listed in the same order as the areas described in the previous section on exploration and control.

Arterial Injuries

In the suprarenal aortic area, the *celiac axis* can be ligated for bleeding control and better exposure of the aorta if injured. Although collateral supply to the intestine is usually excellent in most trauma patients, there is a substantial risk for gallbladder necrosis. Therefore, celiac axis ligation is recommended primarily in multitrauma high-risk patients in whom portal blood flow is intact. Aortic injuries at this level are repaired by 3-0 or 4-0 sutures. The first 3–4 cm of *SMA* accessible through suprarenal exposure must be repaired if injured. The middle portion can be ligated provided that blood flow through the celiac axis and inferior mesenteric artery is intact. Accordingly, ligating both the celiac axis and the SMA leads to extensive necrosis and should not be done. A bypass from the infrarenal aorta using saphenous vein to the distal SMA is a good option if feasible. The *left renal artery* should also be mended if possible; 5-0 sutures are often suitable, and patches are used liberally for both renal artery and SMA repair. If the left renal artery is severely damaged, nephrectomy is an option to consider when the right kidney is functioning properly.

The *right renal artery* is encountered during exposure of the right infrarenal vena cava. As for the left renal artery, repair is advisable. Injuries to the distal SMA can be treated by ligature if repair is not easy.

Repair of the *infrarenal aorta* is accomplished by suture or graft interposition. For thrombosis occurring after blunt trauma, it is important to remember to ensure that the vessel wall is in good condition before suturing the anastomosis. If injured, the *inferior mesenteric artery* is ligated as close to the aorta as possible. *Common iliac arteries* should be repaired using 5-0 sutures or graft interposition. If either one of these vessels is ligated, amputation rates up to 50% have been reported. Also, the *external iliac arteries* should be repaired, but the *internal iliac arteries* can be ligated. Interrupting blood flow through one of the external iliac arteries leads to almost the same amputation rate as ligating the common iliac arteries. Proximal ligature followed by a femorofemoral bypass is a good alternative for repairing unilateral iliac artery injuries.

Injuries to the *common hepatic artery* in the portal triad do not need to be repaired if portal vein flow is adequate and there is no apparent liver damage. If the *proper hepatic artery* is ligated, the gallbladder may become gangrenous and should be excised liberally. If possible, lacerations in the proper hepatic artery should be sutured, but the artery must be separated from the portal vein and the common bile duct to avoid injuries to these structures. *Splenic and gastric arteries* can be ligated without morbidity.

Venous Injuries

In general, venous injuries are more difficult to manage than arterial ones. There are several reasons for this. It is more difficult to expose and repair vein injuries due to their thin and fragile walls. Distal control is also more difficult to achieve. While arterial backbleeding often is sparse when the patient is in shock, distal bleeding from injured veins increases after proximal control. For surgeons without experience in venous surgery, the consequence is that it is difficult to repair major venous injuries. Fortunately, many veins can be ligated in difficult situations.

The *left renal vein* encountered during suprarenal aortic exposure can be ligated, preferably as close to vena cava as possible to allow alternative outflow through collaterals. Injured veins around the celiac axis can also be ligated. If possible, the proximal *superior mesenteric vein* should be repaired. This vein lies in close connection to the SMA. Control is achieved by manual or rubberband occlusion while suturing the defect. If repair is not possible, ligation leads to venous congestion of the intestine. In general, this is quite well tolerated, and the patient usually survives. However, if the patient becomes hypotensive in the postoperative period, it may be fatal.

Infrahepatic vena cava injuries should be repaired if possible. Interrupted 4-0 sutures can be used for most lacerations. For stab wounds penetrating both the ventral and dorsal part of the vein, access for repair includes extending the anterior opening to be able to close the hole on the dorsal side from the inside. Alternatively, the vena cava is dissected free and the lumbar branches secured and rolled over to expose the wound for suturing. (See Fig. 5.4.)

Small dorsal vena cava injuries not actively bleeding can be observed. In multiply injured patients in bad condition, ligation rather than repair may be preferable. This leads to leg swelling in the postoperative period but is usually well tolerated. No effort should be spared to repair the *right renal vein* if injured because, in contrast to the *left* side, collateral venous outflow is essentially lacking. If the vein must be ligated in difficult situations, right-sided nephrectomy is warranted. Also, the distal parts of the superficial mesenteric vein should be repaired if straightforward. *Portal vein* injuries are taken care of by venoraphy or graft interposition using 5-0 sutures if reasonably easy. Portacaval shunts have also been constructed to repair injuries to the portal vein. It the patient is hypotensive and hypothermic with extensive injuries, it is wise to ligate the portal vein. In most patient series, this maneuver is reported to be associated with survival and low postoperative portal hypertension rates.

NOTE
Repair of the right renal vein is important to save renal function on this side.

Suspected injuries to the *retrohepatic vena cava* area should be packed, and this is often sufficient for permanent bleeding control. Repair of injuries to the vena cava behind the liver and the few centimeters of the right and left hepatic veins outside it requires total vascular control as described previously. A few successful cases have been reported in the literature. To facilitate repair, one branch from the *hepatic vein* can be ligated without morbidity. If the total venous outflow is compromised by interruption of the entire hepatic vein, lobectomy may be necessary. Clips can control caudate veins behind the liver. Anecdotally, retrohepatic caval injuries have been repaired through a liver injury separating the lobes. Final access to the cava may then be achieved by separating parts of any remaining liver tissue using the "finger fracture" technique.

Damaged *common iliac veins* and the first parts of the *vena cava* are difficult to expose for repair. The aortic bifurcation and the common iliac arteries must be freed entirely to allow mobilization and control of the veins. This includes division of lumbar arteries and the sacral artery. As mentioned, temporary division of the left iliac artery is often required to provide exposure of the left iliac vein. Polypropylene suture, 5-0, is appropriate for repair. A good option for multiply injured patients

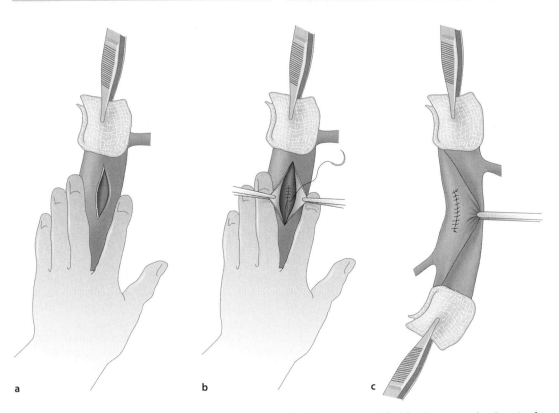

a   b   c

Fig. 5.4. a Manual control of bleeding from an injury in the ventral wall of vena cava. **b** Repair of the dorsal injury of the vena cava through an anterior injury after stabbing through both walls. Note that no vascular clamps are used for bleeding control. **c** Repair of a dorsal injury after separation and rotation of the vena cava

in shock is ligation of the distal vena cava or the common iliac vein.

Distal *iliac vein* injuries should be repaired. Ligation of the *internal iliac vein* often facilitates release of the external iliac vein and provides better exposure of the injured site. In high-risk patients if repair is not feasible, a good option is ligation. Unfortunately, distal control of internal iliac veins is difficult. Often the best way is to use compression with a sponge-stick for distal control while suturing the lacerations. It is important to reduce bleeding by closing the hole even if narrowing or obstruction of the vein is the final result.

Final Vascular Repair After "Damage Control"

With any luck the patient will have improved hemodynamically after a period of resuscitation in the intensive care unit and does not have hypothermia, coagulopathy, or acidosis and is more stable. He or she is then returned to the operating room for final repair of vascular and other injuries. When arterial injury is suspected at the primary operation, angiography should be performed first to identify and provide information before repair. This can take place any time between a few hours to 10 days after the primary operation. The second operation consists of meticulous exploration of injured areas still bleeding, including hematomas and cavities. Any recurrent bleeding is controlled and repaired as outlined previously. Shunted vessel segments must also be controlled and repaired. It is difficult to give well-founded advice regarding final repair of previously ligated vessels. A suggestion is to consider the hepatic artery and the SMA for secondary repair. It is usually not worthwhile to try to mend ligated veins. After final repair of organ and intestinal injuries, the packs are removed and the abdomen closed. It is not uncommon that renewed hemorrhage necessitates repacking and a second period in the intensive care unit. It the literature this is reported to happen in up to 10% of patients.

5.5.2.5 Finishing the Operation

After vascular repair, other injuries are taken care of. For a detailed description, we recommend trauma textbooks. If the peritoneal cavity is contaminated, careful cleansing using warmed fluids is recommended. If possible, vascular anastomoses should be covered with tissue. If the SMA and proximal aorta are injured, it is important to assess the viability of the intestine before closing the abdomen. Sites of vessel repair should also be checked one more time. Minor – and even quite substantial – bleeding from such areas can be managed by hemostatic adjuvant therapy, such as local application of fibrin glue or gel (page 189).

5.5.3 Endovascular Treatment

Endoluminal aortic stent-graft repair has become a possible option for blunt aortic injuries missed during initial exploration, especially in the thoracic part of the aorta. In some of cases reported in the literature, the injured aortic site causing dissection was treated by fenestration and stent placement. Other patients had stable hematomas that were examined with CT and found to involve partial aortic occlusion. Also, injuries in the common iliac artery caused by pelvic fracture have been treated by stent-grafts. In one series, a few patients had iliac artery occlusions that were passed with a guide wire and then successfully treated with a covered stent. This approach may be particularly tempting when conventional repair is not possible due to associated injuries and pelvic hematoma. Angiography and subsequent embolization of branches from the internal iliac artery for bleeding due to pelvic fracture is successful in many instances. One should remember that in up to 5% of patients, gluteal muscle necrosis occurs after such branch embolization.

Blunt and penetrating renal trauma can also be managed by endovascular methods. Selective embolization of bleeding renal artery branches is often successful. Isolated dissection and subsequent thrombosis of a renal artery after blunt trauma diagnosed during early management is preferably treated by angioplasty and stenting, providing that angiography facilities are available and that such management does not delay final treatment.

Blunt abdominal trauma causing splenic injury can also be treated by endovascular embolization. In most published patient series, CT has been insufficient for selecting patients for endovascular therapy, and diagnostic angiography is recommended to rule out this possibility. High-quality CT angiography, however, readily identifies such lesions. Observed patients who continue to require fluids and blood because of the organ injury should undergo arteriography to rule out treatable injuries. Examples are intraperitoneal or intraparenchymal contrast extravasation and vessel truncation, which are all amenable to embolization. Treatment then consists of selective catheterization and injection of microcoils.

The late consequences of abdominal vascular injuries – pseudoaneurysm and arteriovenous fistula – can also be treated by endovascular methods in most locations. To our knowledge, there are no reports of successful endovascular treatment of venous injuries in the abdomen.

5.5.4 Management After Treatment

It is obvious that patients with abdominal vascular injuries have a high risk for developing serious complications in the postoperative period. Hypotension due to continued blood loss is common, and reoperation should be employed liberally. Visceral and leg ischemia may also occur due to ligated or thrombosed repaired vessel segments. The abdominal appearance and leg perfusion must therefore be monitored meticulously in the postoperative period. Examination should, besides abdominal palpation, consist of a rectal examination and inspection of the nasogastric tube to check for blood. Renal artery thrombosis may manifest as flank pain and a temporary rise in serum creatinine. Occasionally, emergency nephrectomy is necessary in the postoperative period due to pain or a very high blood pressure.

As mentioned before, it is extremely important to keep the blood pressure at adequate levels if the intestinal blood supply is compromised by a deliberate ligation during exploration. Extra careful cardiac monitoring, fluid resuscitation, and pharmacological blood pressure adjustment are warranted. If intestinal ischemia is suspected, immediate relaparotomy is indicated.

Swelling after vein ligation or thrombosis of a repaired major vein segment is also a common problem. The measures recommended to minimize this problem are supplying the patient with compression stockings and infusing dextran to optimize the rheology of the blood. Furthermore, as soon as the patient is hemodynamically stable, standardized heparinization should be initiated. Patients with repaired injuries in the portal vein and the superior mesenteric vein may also develop portal hypertension and hepatic failure.

Antibiotics should be continued postoperatively. Patients arriving in shock are prone to infection, especially if intestinal perforation is part of the trauma spectrum. Careful monitoring of infection signs is necessary, and CT examination is indicated if intraabdominal infection is suspected.

5.6 Results and Outcome

Outcome after abdominal vascular trauma is strongly related to whether shock is present at arrival. The time elapsing from the trauma to the patient's arrival at the hospital is important. For example, few patients survived penetrating abdominal vascular trauma during World War II, whereas 42% did during the Vietnam War. In series from civilian life looking at survival of patients with aortic or vena cava injuries arriving alive to the hospital, around half have been reported to survive. Besides shock, free bleeding in the peritoneal cavity and suprarenal location of the injury are risk factors for poor outcome. Survival rates after blunt trauma are around 75% in the literature. Observational studies including 200 patients or more list suprarenal or juxtarenal aortic injuries, retrohepatic and hepatic vein injuries, and portal vein injuries as associated with the highest mortality.

It is more difficult to find data on survival rates for isolated injuries to a specific vessel. One report of isolated arterial injuries or those combined with other arterial injuries in the abdomen found mor-

tality to range from 30% for hepatic artery to 80% for aortic injuries. The mortality for renal, iliac, and SMA injuries was around 50–60%.

Abdominal venous trauma is also associated with high mortality due to exsanguination. Overall, mortality ranges from 30–70%. The worst results come from patient series of retrohepatic vena cava injuries, reporting a mortality of over 90%. Also, portal vein and superior mesenteric vein injuries lead to substantial mortality. In one study, 30% died after lateral repair of the portal vein and 78% after ligation of this vessel. The latter procedure, however, was performed in more severely injured patients with more associated injuries. Another study reported only 20% mortality after portal vein ligation. In patients with only venous injuries or in combination with other venous trauma, the mortality rates were 75% for inferior vena cava injury, 72% for portal vein injury, 56% for renal vein injury, and 44% for iliac vein injury.

5.7 Iatrogenic Vascular Injuries in the Abdomen

It is not uncommon that vessels are injured during abdominal surgery for malignancy or other procedures. Some procedures are particularly prone to cause injury to abdominal vessels. A discussion on some of these follows below. The principles of repair are essentially the same as for traumatic injury caused by accidents or violence.

5.7.1 Laparoscopic Injuries

Trocars used for laparoscopic access frequently cause injury to major blood vessels in the abdomen. When the aorta or vena cava is injured, outcome may even be fatal. The insufflation needle may also cause severe injuries. Injury is more common in thin patients who have previously undergone abdominal operations and in patients in whom a blind technique for inserting the trocar is used. When blood returns through the trocar or needle, a severe injury should be suspected. Another situation indicating vascular injury occurs when the patient becomes hypotensive or when the abdomen swells rapidly before the gas is insufflated. If the aorta or iliac arteries are injured conversion to an open operation by a midline incision to achieve proximal control is necessary to save the patient. Lateral repair or, occasionally, graft interposition is usually possible for final repair.

Vascular injury may also occur during the procedure itself, during dissection by careless handling of the instruments and occasionally by retractors. Because visualization is hampered by the bleeding, open repair is always recommended.

■ 5.7.2 Iliac Arteries and Veins During Surgery for Malignancies in the Pelvis

Distortion of the pelvic anatomy is common in malignant disease. Therefore, the surgical procedures for tumor removal are often difficult, and injuries, especially to veins, are sometimes unavoidable to make radical excision possible. The injury becomes obvious by the bleeding, and because it is usually veins that are injured, control is accomplished by compression. Definitive repair is often more difficult. If major veins such as the iliacs are damaged, suturing of the hole is possible during inflow and outflow control, either manually or by sponge-sticks. It is necessary to reduce bleeding sufficiently so that the hole can be visualized adequately for repair. Often, however, it is the internal iliac or, rather, branches from this vein that bleed. Sufficient control for repair is then almost impossible to achieve, and attempts to apply "blind" sutures often make the bleeding worse. When the bleeding is moderate, simple compression sometimes permanently stops it. If not, fibrin glue should be applied, followed by another period of manual compression. If surgical repair is impossible and compression and local therapies have been tried unsuccessfully, the only way to reduce the bleeding might be to ligate the internal iliac arteries. Before this measure, the surgeon must check that the patient's coagulation status is as optimal as possible. The risk that this will cause gluteal muscle necrosis is considerable, but it may occasionally be indicated. If the patient's condition is stable enough and the operating room is equipped for combined surgical and endovascular procedures, allowing angiography to identify the bleeding site and selective coiling bleeding vessel branches, this risk can be reduced considerably.

In an ultimate situation the bleeding pelvic area can be packed with an intestinal bag filled with a number of swabs tied together. The abdominal wall is closed allowing the opening of the plastic bag with the end of the swabs to protrude. The patient is then brought to the ICU for "damage control" and the swabs and the plastic bag subsequently removed one or two days later.

■ 5.7.3 Iliac Artery Injuries During Endovascular Procedures

Perforation and dissection of the common and external iliac arteries are common during endovascular procedures, but this rarely leads to severe bleeding. Most of the time, complications can be managed by immediate stenting or stent-graft repair. Occasionally the bleeding will continue or is not discovered during the procedure, and the patient displays symptoms a few hours after the procedure. Often, he or she complains of severe abdominal pain in the flank of the injured side. The abdomen is positive for tenderness, and the patient's general condition shows signs of ongoing bleeding. If one is in doubt, a CT can confirm the diagnosis, but the diagnosis is usually obvious. Most patients are unstable and should be taken to the operating room for immediate repair. A midline incision is then recommended because it enables proximal control of the distal aorta if necessary. The hematoma makes it difficult to identify the injury site, and a bypass followed by ligation of the common iliac artery is the best way to treat it. Besides an iliofemoral bypass, one good option is to perform a femorofemoral bypass. If the artery is stented all the way up to the aortic bifurcation, it is almost impossible to ligate it or to find a spot for inflow of a bypass. Therefore, the procedure occasionally requires a bypass from the aorta and division of the iliac artery.

■ 5.7.4 Iatrogenic Injuries During Orthopedic Procedures

Lumbar disc surgery is reported to cause aortic or common iliac artery injury in 1–5 out of 10,000 operations. The mechanism is laceration caused by the special instruments used for excising the herniated disc. This injury generally presents as a substantial bleeding in the wound, with an associated systemic hypotension. Occasionally, the diagnosis becomes apparent after the procedure when signs of shock develop during the first postoperative hours. Even more common is that an arteriovenous fistula or pseudoaneurysm is found, which is diagnosed any time from a few hours after the procedure to several years postoperatively. Findings suggesting such injuries are, in descending order of frequency, bruits, heart failure, abdominal pain, and hypotension. The disc level where the surgery is performed determines which vessel becomes injured. At the L4–L5 and L5–S1 levels, the common iliac artery and vein are injured. Higher up, the aorta and vena cava are at risk.

For emergency repair, a midline incision for exposure is needed, and the same principles are applicable as for other types of trauma: lateral repair, patching, or graft insertion. Arteriovenous fistulas and pseudoaneurysms may also be treated using endovascular methods.

During hip arthroplasty, the external iliac vessels or the common femoral artery may be injured. While uncommon at primary procedures, it happens more often during revisions because of the need to remove previous prosthetic material and the anatomical alterations caused by previous surgery. The left side is more often injured. The mechanism is sometimes direct lacerations by acetabular screws, dissection, or traction injury, but more common is cement destruction of the vessels. Arterial repair is performed after obtaining proximal control of the common iliac artery. Usually, a "hockey-stick" incision is sufficient to obtain exposure. Destroyed vessel segments by cement need graft interposition or a bypass.

Further Reading

Baker WE, Wassermann J. Unsuspected vascular trauma: blunt arterial injuries. Emerg Med Clin North Am 2004; 22(4):1081–1098

Brown CV, Velmahos GC, Neville AL, et al. Hemodynamically "stable" patients with peritonitis after penetrating abdominal trauma: identifying those who are bleeding. Arch Surg. 2005; 140(8):767–772

Fuller J, Ashar BS, Carey-Corrado J. Trocar-associated injuries and fatalities: an analysis of 1399 reports to the FDA. J Minim Invasive Gynecol 2005; 12(4):302–307

Gupta N, Solomon H, Fairchild R, et al. Management and outcome of patients with combined bile duct and hepatic artery injuries. Arch Surg 1998; 133(2):176–181

Lee JT, Bongard FS. Iliac vessel injuries. Surg Clin North Am 2002; 82(1):21–48

Malhotra AK, Latifi R, Fabian TC, et al. Multiplicity of solid organ injury: influence on management and outcomes after blunt abdominal trauma. J Trauma 2003; 54(5):925–929

Nicholas JM, Rix EP, Easley KA, et al. Changing patterns in the management of penetrating abdominal trauma: the more things change, the more they stay the same. J Trauma 2003; 55(6):1095–1108; discussion 1108–110

Parks RW, Chrysos E, Diamond T. Management of liver trauma. Br J Surg 1999; 86(9):1121–1135

Smith SR. Traumatic retroperitoneal venous haemorrhage. Br J Surg 1988; 75(7):632–636

Sugrue M, D'Amours SK, Joshipura M. Damage control surgery and the abdomen. Injury 2004; 35(7):642–648

Weber S, Murphy MM, Pitzer ME, et al. Management of retrohepatic venous injuries with atrial caval shunts. AORN J 199664(3):376–377, 380–382

Acute Intestinal Ischemia

6

CONTENTS

■ 6.1 Summary

- Triad of symptoms
  1. History of embolization
  2. Pain out of proportion
  3. Intestinal emptying
- Urgent management is essential: rehydration, angiography and laparotomy
- If arterial obstruction – aggressive surgical treatment
- If venous obstruction – restrictive with surgical treatment
- Embolectomy if jejunum is normal

■ 6.2 Background

Acute intestinal ischemia is often a fatal disease, and many patients with this disorder will die regardless of treatment. Increased awareness and rapid management can improve this pessimistic course. Using wide definition acute intestinal ischemia is hypoxia of the small intestinal wall due to a sudden decrease of perfusion caused by emboli or arterial or venous thrombosis. The symptoms are not specific, and the diagnosis is regularly established at laparotomy late in the course when peritonitis has developed. With rapid and efficient management, including an aggressive diagnostic work-up, the number of successful embolectomies can increase and the need for extensive intestinal resections can be diminished. The diagnosis must be established early in the course of the disease. A high level of clinical suspicion when evaluating acute abdominal pain, prompt management in the emergency department, and early angiography or laparotomy is required to achieve this.

6.2.1 Magnitude of the Problem and Patient Characteristics

Even if patients with acute intestinal ischemia are usually admitted and treated by general surgeons, cooperation with a vascular surgeon may be a possible way to improve treatment results. Vascular surgeons contribute with their experience of angiography as well as with operations in the area around the superior mesenteric artery (SMA).

The disease is relatively uncommon. Among all patients arriving in the emergency department because of abdominal pain, 0.5 % have acute intestinal ischemia. The true incidence is probably higher because patients can be suspected to die from intestinal ischemia without an established diagnosis. The relatively low incidence in combination with the imprecise symptoms and moderate findings at physical examination early in the course of the disease contribute to the bad prognosis. In observational studies the 30-day mortality is 60–85% for patients who are not treated surgically with the diagnosis established by angiography or physical examination. One more factor contributing to the poor prognosis is that this category of patients consists of elderly who have complicating diseases such as chronic obstructive pulmonary disease and generalized arteriosclerosis, including coronary disease. In most studies, the mean patient age is around 70 years. Two-thirds of the patients are female.

Intestinal ischemia secondary to mesenteric venous thrombosis is associated with another group of patients and has a significantly better prognosis. The 30-day mortality is around 30%. Five to 15% of all cases presenting with intestinal ischemia are caused by venous thrombosis.

6.3 Pathophysiology

The main blood supply to the small intestine comes from the SMA, which also perfuses the first half of the colon. The inferior mesenteric artery and branches from the internal iliac arteries supply the distal part of colon and rectum. This double blood supply and an extensive collateral network explain why occlusion of the inferior mesenteric artery seldom causes severe ischemia in the distal colon. Primary ischemia of the colon is

unusual and is further discussed in Chapter 12 on complications in vascular surgery. The rest of this chapter will deal with acute ischemia of the small intestine.

NOTE
Occlusion of the SMA has devastating effects on the perfusion of the intestine.

Because almost the entire small intestine gets its blood supply from one single artery, a sudden occlusion of this vessel has major consequences. The initial response is spasm and vigorous contraction. Because of its high metabolic activity 80% of the blood supply to the intestine is consumed by the mucosa. This explains why the mucosa is damaged before the rest of the intestinal wall is. The cells at the tip of the villi are most sensitive and die first. Under the microscope, ischemic changes can be seen in the mucosa within 30 min after occlusion. Patients with SMA occlusion will, very early after onset, vomit and have diarrhea and abdominal pain. Occasionally they have blood in their stools. Granulocytes are also activated early, and oxidants and proteolytic enzymes affect the intestine. Hypotension develops as the next step in the course of the disease and contributes to further ischemic damage of the intestinal wall. This is followed by diffuse necrosis in the mucosa that spreads to the submucosal layer and finally extends through the entire intestinal wall. The result is transmural infarction and local peritonitis. The intestine then may perforate, and the patient develops general peritonitis. Metabolic acidosis, dehydration, anuria, and multiple organ failure could be the end result.

The main etiology of acute intestinal ischemia is embolization or thrombosis of the SMA, both being equally common. In general, an embolus occludes a relatively healthy artery with immediate dramatic consequences as described above, whereas a thrombotic occlusion is preceded by a stenosis, allowing collaterals to develop. The artery may then occlude without causing symptoms or ischemic damage to the intestine.

A less common cause is venous thrombosis. This frequently affects younger patients and typically is secondary to trauma, inflammation, and other diseases in which hypercoagulation is common. It may also be a consequence of congenital coagulation disorders.

Other more unusual causes for acute intestinal ischemia, which are not within the scope of this book, are embolic or thrombotic occlusion of the celiac trunk and the low-flow state nonocclusive intestinal ischemia (NOMI), a result of severe cardiac dysfunction.

6.4 Clinical Presentation

6.4.1 Medical History

In many patients the initial clinical presentation of SMA obstruction is vague, making diagnosis difficult. A triad of symptoms in the patients' medical history should make the surgeon suspicious for acute intestinal ischemia caused by occlusion of the SMA:

1. Severe periumbilical pain ("pain out of proportion")
2. Vomiting and/or diarrhea ("gut-emptying")
3. Possible source of an embolus, or a previous embolization in the medical history.

NOTE

It is important to remember the triad of symptoms associated with occlusion of SMA.

6.4.1.1 Embolism

For a typical patient with embolic occlusion of the SMA, the symptoms include all three elements of the triad. These are then sufficient for determining the diagnosis, as well as for differentiating it from other causes of acute abdominal pain and thrombosis of the same artery. The pain, which often precedes vomiting or diarrhea, is the key symptom. It has a dramatic precipitous onset and is localized in the paraumbilical region. The pain is usually severe and colicky. The expression "pain out of proportion" indicates that there is a discrepancy between the findings in the physical examination of the abdomen and the pain intensity. The pain disappears when the intestine becomes necrotic, which may create a pain-free interval that frequently is misinterpreted as if the patient has improved. The pain returns when the intestine perforates. Ninety-five percent of

Table 6.1. Percentage of patients with symptoms and laboratory findings at the time of admission to the hospital, where the diagnosis acute intestinal ischemia due to arterial occlusion was established later

Symptoms/finding	Frequency
Abdominal pain	100%
Diarrhea or vomiting	84%
Previous embolization/ source of emboli	33%
Blood in stools	25%
Elevated lactate in plasma	90%
Leukocytosis	65%
Metabolic acidosis	60%

these patients have a history of previous cardiac disease, and 30% have had earlier episodes of embolization to other vascular systems (Table 6.1). Embolization is common after acute myocardial infarction, debut of arterial fibrillation, and as a complication of angiography and endovascular treatment.

6.4.1.2 Thrombosis

Thrombosis of the SMA occurs in patients with general arteriosclerosis and a history remarkable for previous manifestations of cardiac and peripheral vascular disease. Sometimes symptoms of chronic intestinal ischemia also are present. The onset of symptoms after acute thrombotic occlusion is more insidious than for embolic disease. The pain is usually constant and progressive over several hours but is otherwise similar to what has been described for embolism. (See Table 6.2.)

For thrombosis of the mesenteric vein, the duration of symptoms is commonly several days and the symptoms are even more imprecise than for arterial occlusion. The pain is less pronounced but is present to some degree in 90% of patients. Fever is also a common sign. Eighty-five percent of patients have a history of hypercoagulation disorders such as deep venous thrombosis or have had other diseases or risk factors predisposing them to thrombosis. Examples include pregnancy, oral contraceptive use, malignancy, inflammatory diseases, portal hypertension, and trauma.

Table 6.2. Differentiation between causes of intestinal ischemia (*DVT* deep vein thrombosis)

	Arterial embolism	Arterial thrombosis	Venous thrombosis
Older	+	+	–
Younger	–	–	+
Previous symptoms of chronic intestinal ischemia	–	+	–
Previous DVT	–	–	+
Possible source emboli	+	–	–
Sudden onset	+	–	–
Insidious onset	–	+	+

6.4.2 Physical Examination

Findings at physical examination in acute intestinal ischemia can be vague and difficult to interpret. It is still, however, very important to carefully examine the patient. The examination reveals signs of arteriosclerosis – carotid bruits, heart murmur, and so on – as well as sources of embolus. Abdominal examination findings are the basis for emergency management. For instance, without signs of peritonitis, a patient should not undergo laparotomy when venous thrombosis is the suspected diagnosis. A patient with arterial occlusion, however, needs surgery before peritonitis evolves.

The abdominal findings vary with the time point during the course of the illness when the patient is examined. Anything from normal findings to general peritonitis may be found. In early stages, a slight tenderness and amplified bowel sounds are common findings, but when peritonitis is established, tenderness with muscular guarding and a lack of bowel sounds due to paralysis are found. Abdominal distension is a very late sign in the course of the disease. The examination should also assess the patient's general condition, including possible dehydration.

6.5 Diagnostics

For the majority of patients with the triad of symptoms described the need for further diagnostic work-up is limited and immediate laparotomy is indicated. Laboratory tests can support the diagnosis but should not delay management and treatment. The only radiologic examination that is warranted, besides computed tomography (CT) for diagnosing suspected venous thrombosis, is angiography and perhaps plain x-ray. The resources and expertise available in the hospital should also influence the decision of whether any further investigations or tests are performed.

6.5.1 Laboratory Tests

The leukocyte count is elevated early in the disease course. Together with the clinical triad, a leukocyte count higher than $15 \times 10^9/l$ is pathognomonic for acute intestinal ischemia. Values above normal for serum lactate and D-dimer have also been suggested as prognostic markers for patients who need surgery. A lactate concentration exceeding 2.6 mmol/l is considered to have a high sensitivity (90–100%) for acute mesenteric ischemia, meaning that only one patient in 10 with intestinal ischemia has a value <2.6 mmol/l and is at risk to be missed by this test. The specificity with this cut-off value, however, is rather low (around 40%). Overall, provided that shock, diabetes, severe renal insufficiency, and pancreatitis have been ruled out, an elevated plasma lactate indicates that the patient has a disease very likely to be acute intestinal ischemia, and that the patient definitely has a disease that needs surgery. More pronounced leukocytosis and elevated hemoglobin and hematocrit values are secondary to plasma losses in the injured intestine. Later, when the intestinal wall becomes necrotic and blood leaks into the intestinal lumen, hemoglobin and hematocrit decrease.

Metabolic acidosis also occurs late in the course of the disease, and as a diagnostic test it has no value. The acid-base balance, however, needs to be monitored and corrected continuously during the course of treatment as a general measure.

6.5.2 Angiography

In hospitals where angiography is available 24 h a day and can be performed rapidly, it is recommended before laparotomy for most patients suspected of having this disease. Exceptions are patients with peritonitis. Angiography can possibly be preceded by a plain x-ray to exclude free gas in the abdomen. Besides establishing the diagnosis, angiography is also helpful for separating the different etiologies for acute intestinal ischemia:

1. *Embolization to the SMA:* Typically, this appears as a "meniscus" occlusion located 5–7 cm out in the SMA, which has its first branches open and filled with contrast. Such emboli are usually possible to extract by simple embolectomy.

2. *Arterial thrombosis* in previously atherosclerotic arteries: On the films an occlusion of the SMA is found approximately 1–2 cm from its origin and no distal branches are filled with contrast. Sometimes the patient can then be reconstructed with a bypass from the aorta. In many circumstances, however, it is wise to avoid laparotomy if the contrast does not reach any part of the SMA. Total SMA thrombosis is rarely curable by reconstructive vascular surgery. Thrombolysis may then be an option if a guide wire can be inserted into the artery.

3. *Venous thrombosis or NOMI:* If the branches from the SMA can be followed some distance out in the mesentery – more than 10 cm from the origin – and the contrast is moving slowly, the finding indicates a state of threatening infarction without arterial occlusion. This can be due to either venous thrombosis or NOMI. Laparotomy is not indicated in such patients.

NOTE

Emergency angiography is often helpful for diagnosing and managing acute intestinal ischemia.

The surgeon is responsible for making sure that angiography will not cause an unacceptable delay in the management process. It should be performed with close observation of the patient, including continuous monitoring of vital signs and abdominal status. In hospitals without available angiography, management has to be based on clinical findings only. If this investigation resource is available, however, and the department has experience with emergency angiography, it is recommended.

TECHNICAL TIPS
The technique for angiography in acute mesenteric ischemia

1. Scrub and dress for groin puncture.
2. Shoot one plain frontal and one lateral x-ray (to exclude free gas).
3. Puncture the femoral artery. Insert a guide wire and any angiography catheter. Place the tip at the level of the first lumbar vertebra.
4. Withdraw the guide wire and rapidly inject by hand 10 ml of x-ray contrast. Images are first obtained in the frontal plane to visualize embolization to the SMA.
5. Repeat with the lateral projection (this is always necessary to diagnose thrombosis when the SMA is occluded at the origin).
6. Consider injecting papaverine (1–2 ml of 40 mg/ml) through the catheter, preferably after its tip has been placed selectively into the SMA.
7. Pull the catheter and control the puncture site by digital compression.

6.5.3 Other Options

Ultrasound, including determination of flow velocity and color coding (duplex), is often technically difficult to perform because of obscuring intestinal gas and is not recommended for diagnosing acute intestinal ischemia. There are occasional reports in the literature, however, about successful visualization of an occluded SMA that has been helpful for diagnosis. Another possible benefit of an ultrasound examination is to exclude other causes of the patient's symptoms such as renal or gall bladder diseases.

When there is a strong suspicion of venous thrombosis – for example in young patients with a history of hypercoagulation who have mild prolonged symptoms without peritonitis on physical examination – a CT scan with contrast should be performed to establish the diagnosis. The findings on the CT scan that indicate thrombosis are thrombus in the superior mesenteric vein and occasionally in the portal and splenic veins together with splenomegaly. Gas bubbles in these veins may also be found.

6.5.4 Diagnostic Pitfalls

The three main difficulties in diagnosing and managing patients with acute mesenteric ischemia are (1) to suspect the diagnosis, (2) to make the diagnosis fast enough, and (3) to differentiate between thrombotic and embolic etiologies.

Patients with ruptured abdominal aortic aneurysms, a ruptured urinary bladder, hemorrhagic pancreatitis, or a perforated ulcer may also have "pain out of proportion." But their medical history and physical findings are usually sufficient to differentiate between these alternative diagnoses and acute intestinal ischemia. Moreover, for all patients with these diseases, except for pancreatitis, emergency laparotomy is indicated, and a wrong preoperative diagnosis is not so harmful. If not earlier the correct diagnosis can then be established during surgery. Overall, a high level of suspicion and early laparotomy will probably save lives.

While an early diagnosis is essential, the delay caused by performing angiography is often worth the time. Besides establishing the diagnosis and avoiding unnecessary laparotomies, it will also support management decisions during surgery. The relatively low complication rate of angiography also motivates liberal use. It will not negatively affect the management of the few patients suspected to have acute intestinal ischemia who later turn out to have other diseases. Thrombolysis may also be a reasonable treatment option for acute mesenteric ischemia, further supporting an aggressive preoperative diagnostic work-up that includes angiography.

6.6 Management and Treatment

6.6.1 Management Before Treatment

6.6.1.1 In the Emergency Department

Most patients admitted to the emergency department with the described typical combination of physical findings and medical history should undergo immediate angiography and laparotomy. Although patients with only segmental and not transmural ischemia may improve spontaneously because of sufficient collateral blood flow, this is difficult to identify preoperatively. As soon as the operating room has been notified, the following measures can be taken:

1. Place at least one large-bore intravenous (IV) line.
2. Start infusion of fluids. Ringer's acetate is the first option, but dextran is an alternative, especially if venous thrombosis is suspected.
3. Obtain an electrocardiogram.
4. Draw blood for hemoglobin and hematocrit, prothrombin time, partial thromboplastin time, complete blood count, creatinine, sodium, and potassium as well as a sample for blood type and cross-match. Consider ordering a D-dimer as well.
5. Draw arterial blood for acid-base balance, including lactate.
6. Obtain informed consent.
7. Consider administering analgesics (5–10 mg opiate IV).

Early involvement of the anesthesiologist to discuss the patient's condition and optimization of organ function is wise. If time allows, this work-up can be done in the intensive care unit. Any acidosis should be corrected, and blood and plasma infusions are often required. Administration of drugs that reduce blood flow to the intestine should be stopped as soon as possible. Such drugs include digitalis, calcium channel blockers, diuretics, and nonsteroidal anti-inflammatory drugs. When the decision to operate is made the patient should receive analgesics; a suggestion is an opiate 5–20 mg IV. Antibiotics directed against intestinal bacteria, such as a cephalosporin and metronidazole, should also be given preoperatively.

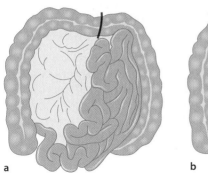 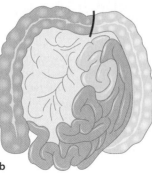

a   b

Fig. 6.1. Acute intestinal ischemia with gangrene. **a** The entire intestine is affected, indicating arterial thrombosis. Surgical treatment possibilities are limited. **b** Ischemic intestinal gangrene but with a viable jejunum and left colon. This typical appearance suggests embolization to the superior mesenteric artery. Embolectomy should be attempted

6.6.2 Operation

The best access is achieved through a long midline incision. The entire intestine should be examined carefully to assess viability (Fig. 6.1). The basic principle is that only parts with transmural necrosis should be resected. It is better to plan for a second-look operation within 24 h than to be very liberal with resection margins. The intestine may appear quite normal at a quick glance, but careful examination often reveals segments with a grayish color and a dull surface, indicating severe ischemia. Viable segments often have pulsations in the distal parts of the mesentery and preserved peristalsis. In addition, a Doppler probe can be helpful in this examination by detecting the presence or absence of arterial flow signals. Healthy segments will have maintained the pink color of a healthy intestine. For a segmental injury, a wedge-shaped excision of the mesentery and the necrotic intestinal segment may be curative and all that is needed for treatment.

6.6.2.1 Embolic Occlusion

If the first part of the jejunum (Fig. 6.1b) looks normal and there are pulsations in the first arterial arcade after the origin of the SMA, embolization is the most probable diagnosis. Under these circumstances embolectomy should be performed before intestinal resection (Technical Tips Box and Fig. 6.2).

6.6.2.2 Arterial Thrombosis

If the entire small intestine and colon are ischemic, the cause is probably arterial thrombosis (Fig. 6.1a). Embolectomy will then not be successful and may even be harmful. If the entire intestine including the right colon is necrotic, the surgeon should consider giving up surgery as treatment and closing the incision. Findings in the preoperative angiography will facilitate this decision.

At least one meter of small intestine is needed for survival. An emergency bypass between the aorta and the SMA is a surgical treatment option for arterial thrombosis. It requires sufficient run-off – often achieved by distal embolectomy and local thrombolysis – verified by intraoperative angiography. The result of such emergency aortomesenteric reconstructions is meager but may nevertheless save a few patients. The technique for this is the same as for chronic disease. It is not covered by this book and we recommend more general vascular surgical manuals for a description.

Chapter 6

TECHNICAL TIPS
Embolectomy of the Superior Mesenteric Artery

Move the transverse colon cranially and identify the SMA by using the fingers to palpate the area ventral to the pancreas behind the superior mesenteric vein. This is facilitated by holding the mesenteric root between the thumb and the fingers. Expose the artery by incising the dorsal peritoneum longitudinally just over the area where the pulse is lost (Fig. 6.2).

This sometimes requires partial division of the ligament of Treitz as well as inferior mobilization of the 4th portion of the duodenum. Apply vessel loops above and below the site of the intended arteriotomy. At least 4–5 cm needs to be exposed. Administer 5,000 units of heparin IV, clamp the artery as close to the aorta as possible, and make a transverse arteriotomy distal to the clamp. Perform embolectomy with a #4 Fogarty catheter. Start proximally while controlling bleeding through the arteriotomy using the vessel loop and a finger. Inflow is usually quite vigorous, and it is important to not cause unnecessary bleeding. Continue distally towards the intestine with same catheter. A #3 catheter is occasionally needed to reach all the way out to the periphery. If the diagnosis is correct, an embolus with a secondary thrombus is extracted, and the backflow is brisk. If not, try a second time with the catheter directed manually into the branches. Inject 2–4 ml of papaverine through a catheter into the SMA. If the backbleeding is inadequate, try to instill the same amount of rtPA into the distal branches. Close the artery with interrupted 6-0 prolene sutures. Place the intestine in its normal position and check the final result by palpating distal pulses and inspecting the intestine. If the viability of the intestine is uncertain, wait 20–30 min before deciding on what parts to remove. Finish the operation by resecting nonviable parts as needed and close the abdomen.

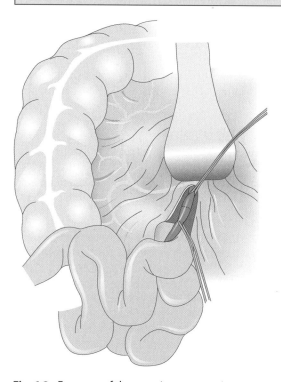

Fig. 6.2. Exposure of the superior mesenteric artery for embolectomy through an incision in the posterior peritoneum

If the intestine not is totally necrotic, it is sensible to wait for 30 min to see whether some segments of the intestine improve so that only a limited resection can be performed.

6.6.2.3 Venous Thrombosis and NOMI

The entire intestine can also be affected in venous thrombosis and NOMI. At laparotomy (which should be avoided if possible), the intestine affected by venous thrombosis will look hyperemic and swollen and may have petechial bleedings in the serosa. If these are found, the operation should be stopped, the abdominal wall closed, and a second-look operation planned. Systemic anticoagulation is the best treatment. At the second-look operation, segments with petechial bleeding might be hard to differentiate from gangrene. Such segments need to be carefully examined to avoid unnecessary resections. Devitalized intestine in segmental venous thromboses, however, should be resected with safe margins. This is different from what is recommended for intestinal ischemia with arterial causes. Venous thrombectomy and thrombolysis have anecdotally been reported, but there is not much evidence that this is beneficial for the patient.

Patients with NOMI may also not be discovered before laparotomy. The intestine then displays the same appearance as for embolic and especially thrombotic obstruction of the main artery. Intraoperative diagnosis relies on pulse palpation and insonation of the distal vascular bed with continuous-wave Doppler. Patients with NOMI have preserved pulses and flow signals – monophasic and throbbing – quite far out distally in the mesentery. These findings together with a typical medical history should be enough to stop the attempt to revascularize the intestine surgically, and the patient needs optimization of cardiac function. The distinction from other arterial causes is difficult, however, and many patients with NOMI are likely to undergo embolectomy by mistake.

6.6.2.4 Endovascular Treatment

At present only limited experience of thrombolytic therapy for acute mesenteric ischemia is available. Until 2003 about 50 cases had been reported in the literature. But the results are promising and the technique may evolve as a primary choice in the future because it fits well with the aggressive work-up required.

The technique for thrombolysis involves groin access and diagnostic angiography as described, preferably with selective catheterization of the SMA and introduction of a guide wire into the thrombus. An end-hole or side-hole catheter is then advanced into the clot and the infusion started by a bolus injection. The catheter is then pulled back somewhat and the continued infusion initiated. The preferable agent is rtPA.

6.6.3 Management After Treatment

While waiting for the second-look operation, the patient should, if possible, be monitored in the intensive care unit. Besides continued fluid losses from the injured intestine, toxic metabolites and proteolytic enzymes are released, which negatively influence heart and lung function. There is also a risk for septicemia because of bacterial translocation. Therefore, rehydration, administration of plasma and blood, and antibiotic treatment are recommended in the early postoperative period. Anticoagulation with heparin should be continued or begun in order to prevent further emboli-

zation and as general prophylaxis against thrombosis, but it probably does not diminish further development of a thrombus in the intestine itself. Because the damaged intestine is prone to bleed, anticoagulation treatment also needs to be monitored carefully.

Reperfusion after a successful embolectomy contributes, as in acute leg ischemia, to morbidity and mortality. The primary damage caused by hypoxia of the intestinal wall is followed by a secondary reperfusion injury. Therefore, patients with acute intestinal ischemia who have been revascularized are possible candidates for adjuvant pharmaceutical treatment to diminish the negative effects on the central organs. The possible substances are often called "scavengers," and examples include superoxide-dismutase, allopurinol, and mannitol. Although all three of these do decrease mortality in animal models, there are presently no clinical trials to support their use in patients.

6.7 Results and Outcome

As mentioned earlier, the mortality associated with acute intestinal ischemia is reported to be very high. Intestinal resection as the only treatment will result in a 30-day mortality of 85–100%. If combined with embolectomy or vascular reconstruction, mortality can be reduced to 55%. In two studies with very positive results, it was proposed that mortality could be reduced to less than 45% if patients are managed very aggressively, with angiography in all patients (except for those with general peritonitis), followed by immediate laparotomy. Ninety percent of the patients who survived in these two studies lost no or less than 30 cm of intestine. The most successful results were observed if the patient reached the operating room within 12 h after the onset of symptoms. Thrombolysis in case series is reported to have excellent results, although the case mix was not comparable to open surgery series, and only a few patients had embolus as the etiology. It is likely that thrombolysis should be attempted as the first option for thrombosis and that this will improve patient survival considerably. Accordingly, the results from most studies favor management and treatment as outlined in this chapter: aggressive diagnostic work-up, liberal indications for laparatomy, embolectomy, and reconstructive vascular surgery.

Further Reading

Angelelli G, Scardapane A, Memeo M, et al. Acute bowel ischemia: CT findings. Eur J Radiol 2004; 50(1):37–47

Burns BJ, Brandt LJ. Intestinal ischemia. Gastroenterol Clin North Am 2003; 32(4):1127–1143

Oldenburg WA, Lau LL, Rodenberg TJ, et al. Acute mesenteric ischemia: a clinical review. Arch Intern Med 2004; 164(10):1054–1062

Schoots IG, Levi MM, Reekers JA, et al. Thrombolytic therapy for acute superior mesenteric artery occlusion. J Vasc Interv Radiol 2005; 16(3):317–329

Williams LF Jr. Mesenteric ischemia. Surg Clin North Am 1988; 68(2):331–353

Ward D, Vernava AM, Kaminski DL, et al. Improved outcome by identification of high-risk nonocclusive mesenteric ischemia, aggressive reexploration, and delayed anastomosis. Am J Surg 1995; 170(6):577–580

Abdominal Aortic Aneurysms

7

CONTENTS

7.1 Summary

- Abdominal aortic aneurysm rupture should always be suspected in men older than 60 years with acute abdominal pain.
- Patients who present with the triad of circulatory shock, abdominal or back pain, and a positive examination for a pulsating mass in the abdomen should immediately be transferred to the operating room for emergency laparotomy.
- Urgent surgery should not be delayed by unnecessary computed tomography or ultrasound scans.

7.2 Background

7.2.1 Magnitude of the Problem

Abdominal aortic aneurysm (AAA) is common. In men older than 60 years the prevalence is 5–10%, which is four times the prevalence in women (Table 7.1). Not more than 1% of men over 60 years of age, however, have an AAA with a diameter around 5 cm, which is the limit at which the risk of rupture is considered motivation for elective operation. The rupture incidence is reported to be 3–15% per 100,000 individuals per year. This means that every surgeon on call as well as emergency department physicians will most likely manage several patients with a ruptured AAA each year. It is possible that the number of patients with ruptured AAAs will decrease in the future because of screening programs. Presently, however, it is still a very common patient type in many countries.

Table 7.1. Prevalence of asymptomatic abdominal aortic aneurysms (>3 cm) in different populations, as determined by ultrasound

Country	Year	N	Population	Prevalence
United Kingdom	1993		Men, 65–75 years	8.4%
United States	1997	73,451	50–79 years	4.7% (men) 1.3% (women)
Netherlands	1998	2,419	Men, 60–80 years	8.1%
Sweden	2001	505	65–75 years	16.9% (men) 3.5% (women)

7.2.2 Pathogenesis

AAA is a dilatation of the aorta caused by degeneration of the elastic components of the arterial wall. The risk for developing AAA is related to atherosclerosis, hypertension, and a genetic predisposition, but its etiology and the pathologic process leading to AAA are unclear. Aneurysms usually originate below the renal arteries and extend down to the aortic bifurcation. The natural course is a gradually increasing dilatation leading to a progressively thinner wall that might end with rupture. The risk of rupture starts to increase exponentially when the aneurysm diameter exceeds 5 cm, but aneurysms of smaller sizes can also rupture. The mortality from a ruptured AAA left untreated is close to 100%, but the length of the process that leads to exsanguination and death varies from minutes to several days. The longer time period involves circumstances when the bleeding is contained within the retroperitoneal space.

7.3 Clinical Presentation

When patients seek medical attention for abdominal or back pain, it is extremely important to always keep the diagnosis of a ruptured AAA in mind.

NOTE

An early correct diagnosis is crucial because the prognosis for patients who are not yet in shock is much better than for those in whom shock has already developed.

7.3.1 Medical History

The classic case of a ruptured AAA is brought to the emergency department by ambulance. Often the patient is a man who experienced immediate onset of severe pain in the upper abdomen with radiation to the back and flanks a few hours earlier. The patient often describes an episode of unconsciousness, dizziness, or sweating when the pain started. Sometimes the family knows that the patient has been previously diagnosed to have an asymptomatic AAA.

7.3.2 Examination

The patient may be circulatory-stable but with positive signs of impending hypovolemic shock: affected consciousness, tachycardia, sweating, and hypotension. A pulsating tender mass is usually found in the epigastrium above the umbilicus. Because the aorta is a dorsal structure in the abdomen, a mass is easy to miss in obese patients. It is also difficult to palpate a pulsating mass when the blood pressure is low because of shock. Accordingly, a pale patient with an increased heart rate and blood pressure <90 mmHg but negative for a pulsating mass may have a ruptured AAA. A distinct local tenderness over the aneurysm is also a common finding. The pain is caused by the retroperitoneal bleeding surrounding the aneurysm. While almost all incipient and already ruptured AAAs are tender, the specificity of this sign is low.

7.3.3 Differential Diagnosis

Patients with a ruptured AAA who are not in shock present with signs that are similar to a variety of other acute diseases in the abdomen or back. To avoid misdiagnosis with conditions that do not require emergency laparotomy, careful examination of the abdominal aorta is important.

Ruptured AAA, or symptomatic aneurysms with incipient rupture, should be included in the discussion about differential diagnosis in all abdominal emergencies, particular in elderly men. Kidney stones located in the ureter, diverticulitis, constipation, intestinal obstruction, pancreatitis, gastric or intestinal perforation, intestinal ischemia, vertebral body compression, and even acute myocardial infarction are all primary diagnoses that can be mixed up with a ruptured AAA. Of course, there is a potential risk of sending a patient home believing that, for example, a ureteral stone has caused the trouble when AAA rupture is the true diagnosis. A significant risk is also related to performing a major operation because of a suspected ruptured AAA in a patient who actually is suffering from an acute myocardial infarction. The only way to avoid this is to keep the AAA diagnosis in mind and to carefully examine the patient.

Another important differential diagnosis is aortic dissection. It is common that a patient will initially have been treated at a smaller healthcare unit or in the emergency department where an ultrasound was performed and misinterpreted as "dissection in an aortic aneurysm." This misunderstanding is caused by the thrombus within the AAA, which can be interpreted as a doubled aortic lumen. There is, however, a clear distinction between rupture and dissection. Rupture is a true burst of the aortic wall with bleeding out from the vessel. Dissection starts with a tear in the inner layer of the vascular wall through which the blood passes and cause a longitudinal separation of the layers, causing a double lumen. Rupture is common in AAA, but dissection is rare (see the information on aortic dissection in Chapter 8).

7.3.4 Clinical Diagnosis

A summary of different clinical presentations of AAA is presented in Table 7.2. These different scenarios can be used in determining the risk for the presence of a ruptured AAA.

NOTE

The presentation of a patient with a ruptured AAA varies, but in most cases a classic triad is found:
- Abdominal pain
- Circulatory instability
- Tender pulsating mass

This combination of symptoms and clinical findings should always be regarded as a ruptured AAA until the opposite is proven.

The purpose of Table 7.2 is to facilitate patient management, and the remaining part of this chapter is largely based on this table. It should be remembered, however, that patients might present with a clinical picture that lies in between the categories.

7.4 Diagnostics

When an aid in detecting AAA is needed, a computed tomography (CT) scan is the first choice for all categories used in Table 7.2. When the suspicion is strong and the risk for sudden deterioration is considered high, the scan should be performed quickly. The responsible surgeon should supervise the procedure so that it can be stopped if necessary and the patient transferred to the operating room immediately. The CT scan should be performed with contrast. The primary questions the scan should answer are as follows: Is there an AAA? Are there signs of rupture? What size is the AAA, and how far proximally and distally does it extend?

NOTE

In the classic case of a ruptured AAA, no diagnostic tools except the physical examination are needed.

Table 7.2. Clinical findings and management of ruptured aortic aneurysms (*AAA* abdominal aortic aneurysm, *OR* operating room, *CT* computed tomography)

Pain	Hemodynamic instability	Pulsating mass	Clinical diagnosis	Measures
Yes	Yes	Yes	Ruptured AAA (classic triad)	Immediate transfer to OR
Yes	Yes	No	Rupture suspected (lack of mass may be due to obesity or low blood pressure)	If history of AAA or signs peritonitis, transfer to OR; Perform ultrasound scan in the OR or CT scan with the surgeon present
Yes	No	Yes	Rupture possible (may have an incipient rupture or an inflammatory aneurysm)	Perform CT scan and consider urgent surgery if diagnosis of AAA is made
Yes	No	No	Rupture unlikely (may have a contained rupture if the patient obese or difficult to palpate)	Perform CT or ultrasound scan

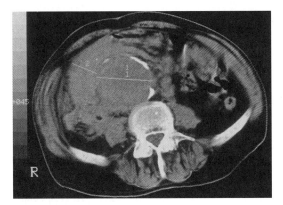

Fig. 7.1. Typical appearance on computed tomography of a ruptured abdominal aortic aneurysm with contrast in lumen, thrombus, calcifications in the wall, and a large retroperitoneal hematoma

To look for anything other than what is mentioned above is unnecessary in an emergency work-up of a patient with a suspected ruptured AAA. The diagnosis made by CT is easy, and typical findings are demonstrated in Fig. 7.1.

Signs of rupture on the scan include a hematoma and contrast that is visible outside the aortic wall retroperitoneally. An early sign of rupture is the presence of contrast in the thrombus and a very thin aortic wall overlying it. The location of the aneurysm in relation to the renal arteries is important for planning an operation but rarely

influences the indication for surgery. It is important to remember that a patient with a diagnosed AAA and pain but with a CT scan showing no signs of rupture needs to be managed as if the patient has impending rupture. Pain may precede rupture, and the scan only answers the question of whether a rupture is already present at the examination. Unfortunately, no signs can predict whether an AAA is going to rupture soon.

There is rarely a place for ultrasound when trying to diagnose a ruptured AAA. Performed in the operating room, it might occasionally be helpful to exclude or verify the presence of an AAA.

When the patient is hemodynamically stable or when the suspicion of rupture is low, the use of additional diagnostic tests to exclude other illnesses is encouraged. Examples of such diseases are pancreatitis and myocardial infarction. These can be verified by electrocardiogram (ECG), a plain abdominal x-ray, a CT scan, ultrasound, or urography as well as by blood tests.

7.5 Management and Treatment

7.5.1 Management Before Treatment

7.5.1.1 Ruptured AAA

If the triad is present the patient needs to be operated without delay caused by preoperative examinations or tests. The time available for making the correct decision regarding patient management is usually limited. The following measures should rapidly be done in the emergency department:

1. Obtain vital signs, medical history, and physical examination.
2. Administer oxygen.
3. Monitor vital signs (heart rate, blood pressure, respiration, SPO_2).
4. Obtain informed consent.
5. Place two large-bore intravenous (IV) lines. Insertion of central lines is time-consuming, and to avoid delays it is better done in the operating room after surgery has started.
6. Start infusion of fluids.
7. Obtain blood for hemoglobin, hematocrit, prothrombin time, partial thromboplastin time, complete blood count, creatinine, blood urea nitrogen, sodium, and potassium, as well as a sample for blood type and cross-match.
8. Catheterize the urinary bladder (this often has to be done in the operating room to gain time) and start recording urine output.
9. Administer analgesics, such as 2–3 mg morphine sulphate IV up to 15 mg, depending on the patient's vital signs, severity of pain, and body weight.
10. Order eight units of packed red blood cells and four of plasma.

The list suggested above may vary among different hospitals. Remember to include pulses, including femoral, popliteal, and pedal, in the physical examination. This is important as a baseline test in case of thromboembolic complications to the legs during surgery. It is also important to be cautious about rehydration and administration of inotropic drugs. The latter should be used only when the patient is in shock and when the low blood pressure threatens to affect cardiac or renal function. The aim should not be to restore the patient's normal blood pressure; a pressure of around 100 mmHg is satisfactory if the patient's vital functions are intact. Hypotension may be an important factor minimizing the bleeding and keeping it contained within the retroperitoneal space. Too intense volume replacement and increased blood pressure may initiate rebleeding.

As soon as possible, the patient should be taken to the operating room and a vascular surgeon contacted. If no surgeon with experience performing AAA procedures is available, consider contacting another hospital and presenting the case to the vascular surgeon there. The patient may then be referred to that hospital or the vascular surgeon could come and perform the procedure if the patient's condition does not allow transport. Even stable patients might start to rebleed at any moment and should therefore not be transported too liberally. If the patient is hemodynamically stable, the start of operation should be delayed until an experienced surgeon is available. However, if there are signs of hemodynamic instability or manifest shock despite treatment, the operation should be initiated. The aim then is to achieve control of the bleeding.

7.5.1.2 Suspected Rupture

The checklist described before is, by and large, also valid when rupture is only suspected.

This category of patients is the most challenging, and generally applicable advice is difficult to give. This category includes patients with a ruptured aneurysm but without a palpable pulsating mass due to obesity and severe hypotension. There are also many other life-threatening conditions that should not be treated with surgery in this group. One such condition is acute myocardial infarction, which also may start with thoracic and abdominal pain and hypotension. Therefore, the surgeon must rapidly decide whether to perform an emergency operation or order diagnostic examinations to verify the diagnosis. In the case of an actual rupture, it is evident that examinations that delay the start of the operation are associated with severe risk. Therefore, every such step should be performed simultaneously with other preoperative measures if possible. For example, ECG is helpful in the diagnosis of myocardial infarction, and ultrasound can verify or exclude the presence of an AAA.

7.5.1.3 Possible Rupture

A tender pulsating mass supports the suspicion of rupture. In a circulatory-stable patient with possible rupture, the following is done in the emergency department:

1. Place an IV line and start a slow infusion of Ringer's acetate.
2. Order an emergency CT scan, with the patient monitored by a nurse.

If the CT scan shows an AAA >5 cm in diameter without signs of rupture and the patient has not displayed hemodynamic instability, the diagnosis impending rupture should be considered. The patient then needs surgery within 24 h. The timing of the operation is based on the patient's condition and the hospital's available resources. While awaiting surgery, patients who need medical treatment to improve cardiac or pulmonary function should receive it. In this category they are also possible candidates for transfer to other hospitals if necessary.

If the patient already has a known aneurysm at admission, the management is also as described above. However, if this known aneurysm has a diameter <4 cm, rupture is unlikely. In such patients the sign of a pulsating mass is also probably lacking. A patient with a known small aneurysm who is in shock should be resuscitated followed by a CT scan. The possibility of cardiogenic shock due to an acute myocardial infarction is a possibility that has to be considered. If cardiac causes have been excluded and the shock is refractory to treatment, laparotomy is advised.

7.5.1.4 Rupture Unlikely

This category of patients should be evaluated with regard to all possible differential diagnoses and managed as any case of "acute abdomen." To rule out or verify AAA a CT scan or ultrasound is performed. The risk for rupture is substantially less for an AAA <5 cm in diameter than for larger aneurysms. The patient should be admitted for observation and worked up considering any other causes of pain, such as kidney stone, pancreatitis, gallstone, perforated duodenal ulcer, perforated intestine, acute myocardial infarction, or vertebral body compression. If the patient does not improve and no other reasonable cause for the pain can be identified, operation of the aneurysm should be considered if it is large.

7.5.2 Operation

7.5.2.1 Starting the Operation

Elevated blood pressure in association with anesthesia induction can accentuate the retroperitoneal bleeding. The patient should therefore be scrubbed and draped and the surgeon ready to start the operation before the patient is anesthetized and intubated. The procedure starts with a long midline incision from the xiphoid process to the pubis. This allows fast and good access to the abdomen. Proximal control of the aorta above the aneurysm is of highest priority. The rest of the operation includes reconstructing the aorta with a straight aortic tube graft or an aortoiliac or aortofemoral bypass graft. The use of autotransfusion of blood, a "cell saver," is recommended. Resuscitation and anesthesia must be monitored closely. The goal is to achieve optimal hemodynamics, with a balance between infused volume and actual, as well as expected, bleeding. The surgeon must realize that it is sometimes necessary to stop the procedure and maintain temporary bleeding control by tamponade or manual compression in order to allow time for the anesthesiologist to compensate for blood and fluid losses. Close contact with the anesthesiologist is important during the entire operation.

7.5.2.2 Exposure and Proximal Control

The conventional technique for exposure and proximal control with a long midline incision and incision of the dorsal peritoneum is recommended. The exposure must sometimes be modified because of bleeding or presence of a hematoma. Infiltration of blood in the tissue surrounding the aneurysm makes it difficult to identify structures such as the mesenteric, renal, and lumbar veins. On the other hand, it often facilitates dissection of the proximal neck by loosening the fibrous tissue adjacent to the aorta.

In a hemodynamically stable patient it is recommended to apply a self-retaining retractor after entering the abdomen. Preferably, a type that is fixed to the table (such as the OmniTrac^{tm}) is used. This facilitates dissection by reducing protruding organs. After incision of the dorsal peritoneum and mobilization of the duodenum to the right, sharp and blunt dissection is used to carefully approach the anterior aspect of the aneurysmal neck (Fig. 7.2).

The correct plane of dissection is reached when the white and smooth surface of the aorta is visualized. An important guide during the dissection through the hematoma is the aortic pulse. Accordingly, a weak pulse due to hypotension makes the dissection more difficult. Exposure of the aneu-

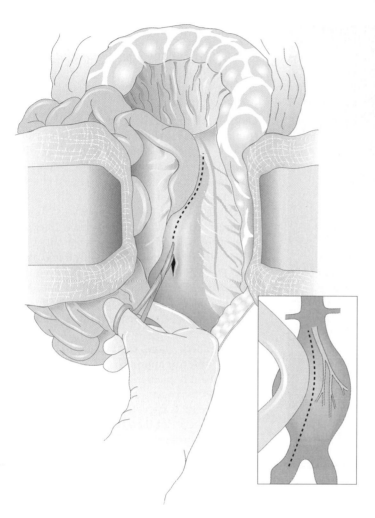

Fig. 7.2. Incision in the posterior peritoneum for exposure of the infrarenal aorta and the neck of an abdominal aortic aneurysm. The incision is placed in the angle between the duodenum and the inferior mesenteric vein, which occasionally has to be divided for good access. A 1–2-cm edge of the peritoneum is left on the duodenum to facilitate restoration of the anatomy at closure

rysmal neck is usually facilitated by the dissection of tissue around the anterior aorta caused by the hematoma. Blunt dissection with a finger behind the aorta in the "friendly triangle" can therefore often be the easiest way to achieve control of the aorta (Fig. 7.3).

When a finger can be pushed behind the aorta, application of the aortic clamp is possible. In this situation an angled Satinsky clamp is suitable. When it is difficult to circumferentially free the aorta, a straight clamp can be applied in an anteroposterior position just inferior to the renal arteries, leaving the aorta adherent dorsally. This often works well, but suturing the anastomosis can be more difficult. The dissection behind the aorta should be performed with great care to avoid damage to the left renal vein, its gonadal branches, and the lumbar veins. Bleeding during this part of the dissection usually emanates from any of these veins and is controlled by ligature, suture, or a local tamponade. Another common source for venous bleeding is the inferior mesenteric vein. It can also be ligated. If profuse bleeding from the ruptured aorta occurs during dissection control can be obtained by several different strategies.

7.5.2.3 Other Options for Proximal Control

There are ways to achieve proximal control of the aorta that fit most situations. The recommendations listed below are ordered according to the probability that they might be needed.

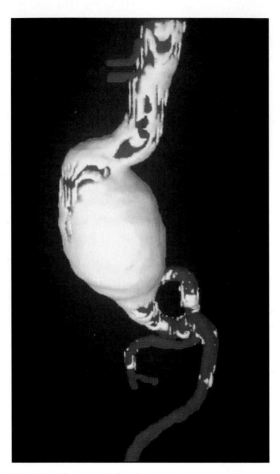

Fig. 7.3. When an abdominal aortic aneurysm is present the anatomy is often changed. The first centimeters of the infrarenal aorta (the neck of the aneurysm) are usually angulated ventrally. The triangular space between the spine, the aneurysm, and its neck is called the "friendly triangle" because its tissue usually allows blunt dissection easily

1. **Manual local compression or "a thumb in the hole"**

   Apply local compression over the rupture with one or several swabs, or try to seal it by putting a finger or thumb into the hole in the aneurysm. This method is convenient when the aneurysm ruptures suddenly during dissection of the neck. It can often be followed by option number two below.

2. **Occlusion with balloon catheter**

   A Foley catheter, size 24-French or larger, is inserted through the hole and the tip is placed proximal to the aneurysmal neck. The balloon is filled with saline until the bleeding diminishes; usually 15–20 ml is sufficient. The remaining bleeding is caused by backbleeding from the distal vascular bed. If it is significant, it has to be controlled before proceeding with dissection of the aneurysmal neck. With this technique the aorta is usually occluded at a suprarenal level and occasionally even higher. When this method is used, the operation should be continued as quickly as possible with exposure of the neck of the aneurysm to allow an aortic clamp to be applied in an infrarenal position. The balloon should then be removed immediately before the clamp is applied. Specially designed balloon catheters for aortic occlusion are also available to facilitate this method of control.

3. **Straight aortic clamp on the neck of the anuerysm – anterior approach**

   If the patient is in severe shock and rapid aortic control is necessary, there is little time for circumferential dissection and exposure. A straight clamp can then be applied as soon as the dorsal peritoneum is divided and the duodenum retracted to the right. It is placed from the ventral portion at the level of the neck. The clamp is positioned by blunt dissection and guided in place by the fingers. The surgeon must be aware of the risk of damaging the vena cava and should also check that the clamp bite includes the entire aortic wall.

4. **Manual compression of the subdiaphragmatic aorta**

   If the rupture is located on the anterior aspect of the aneurysm and there is ongoing significant bleeding within the peritoneal sac, an assistant can achieve temporary proximal control by manual compression of the subdiaphragmatic aorta. This is performed by simply placing the fist against the lesser omentum high up under the xiphoid process and pushing downward and cranially, thereby compressing the aorta against the vertebral column. This gives the surgeon an opportunity to visualize and find the hole, followed by insertion of an occlusive balloon as previously described.

5. **Straight clamp on subdiaphragmatic aorta through the lesser omentum**

   Better control can be achieved by placing an aortic clamp in the subdiaphragmatic position (Fig. 7.4 a–d). The technique is not so easy but is useful when there is a very large hematoma surrounding the neck of the aneurysm, indicating that the rupture is located in that area. In such a case there is considerable risk for uncontrollable bleeding through the rupture when the dorsal peritoneum is opened to expose the aneurysmal neck. To achieve subdiaphragmatic control, the lesser omentum is incised, the aortic hiatus at the diaphragmatic crus is exposed, and the aorta is clamped. The triangular ligament must be divided to allow retraction of the left liver lobe to the right. To avoid damage to the ventricle and esophagus, these organs need to be retracted to the left. Thereafter the muscle fibers in the diaphragmatic crus are divided to allow the straight clamp to be applied in an anteroposterior position. A straight clamp, however, has a tendency to slip off the aorta and cause rebleeding, and repositioning of it is often necessary. This risk is increased if the muscle fibers in the diaphragmatic crus are not cut sufficiently. Great care must be taken to avoid damaging the esophagus and vena cava. As soon as possible, any supraceliac aortic occlusion is replaced by one in an infrarenal position.

6. **Clamping of the thoracic aorta**

   Transthoracic control of the aorta can be used in extreme situations. It is performed through a low left-sided thoracotomy in the 5th–6th intercostal space. The incision starts in the midclavicular line and is extended dorsally as far as possible. After the pleura is incised, the lung is retracted anteriorly and caudally, after which exposure of the thoracic aorta is relatively easy. There are few disturbing surrounding structures. This technique, however, is associated with increased postoperative morbidity and is rarely necessary in the management of ruptured abdominal aortic aneurysms.

7. **Proximal endovascular aortic control**

   In potentially technically challenging and severe cases of ruptured aortic or iliac aneurysms in obese patients or in those with a "hostile" abdomen or traumatic injuries to large intraabdominal, retroperitoneal, or pelvic vessels, it can be advantageous to start the procedure by percutaneously inserting an intraluminal balloon for proximal aortic control (Fig. 7.5). Depending on the location of the injury, this can be done from the groin through the femoral artery or from the arm through the brachial artery. In the former situation, a supporting long introducer left in place is often needed to prevent dislocation by the bloodstream. This procedure requires the surgeon to have experience in endovascular methods or an interventional radiologist to be available for assistance. Briefly the technique is as follows. The brachial artery is punctured with a 12-French introducer. A guide wire is inserted under fluoroscopy with its tip then in the proximal aorta. A 100-cm long catheter with a 46-mm compliant balloon is inserted over the guide wire and connected to a syringe with saline for insufflation. If the patient is in shock the balloon is immediately insufflated by the surgeon for resuscitation. Once positioned such an intraaortic balloon can be temporarily insufflated when needed. This might be a salvaging procedure in many cases of extensive vascular injuries because it controls hemorrhage while allowing dissection of the injured segment. Subsequent application of ordinary vascular clamps can then provide better control. Aortic balloon occlusion can also be valuable in extensive venous injuries in the abdomen or pelvic area because the stopped aortic inflow secondarily leads to diminished venous bleeding.

7.5.2.4 Continuing the Operation

Proximal aortic control usually stabilizes the patient and the operation can proceed as in elective operations for AAA. The iliac arteries are exposed. The aorta and the iliac arteries are clamped, the aneurysm incised, and the thrombus extracted. If there are firm adhesions between the iliac artery and the vein, dissection may be dangerous, potentially causing severe bleeding by injuries to the iliac vein. This can be avoided by using balloon occlusion of the iliac arteries from inside the aneurysm once it has been opened. If there is backbleeding from lumbar arteries, the inferior mesenteric artery, or the median sacral artery, their origins are controlled with 2-0 suture from the inside

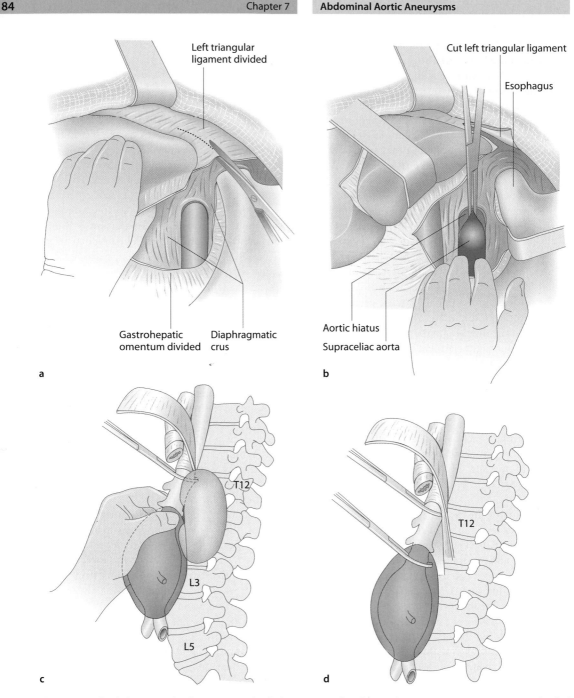

Fig. 7.4. a The left triangular ligament is divided to facilitate exposure of aorta at its diaphragmatic hilus. **b** The gastrohepatic omentum is divided longitudinally, the lesser omental sac entered, and the aorta digitally mobilized at the diaphragmatic crus. **c** After proximal subdiaphragmatic control is achieved by a straight clamp, the posterior peritoneum is divided and the neck of the aneurysm is palpated and digitally dissected, as previously described, through the hematoma. **d** A second clamp is then placed on the neck of the aneurysm and the subdiaphragmatic clamp slowly released

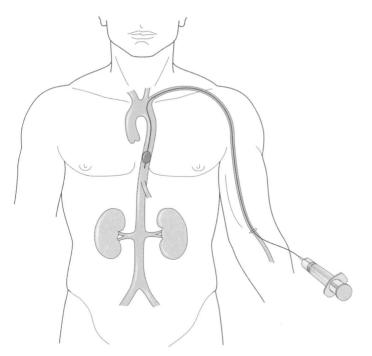

Fig. 7.5. A balloon catheter occluding the aorta at a desired level is inserted through the brachial artery. An alternative is to use a femoral approach with a 16 French 55 cm introducer, supporting the balloon from below

of the aneurysm. Ligature of the inferior mesenteric artery outside the aneurysm should be avoided because this is associated with a certain risk for occlusion of arcade arteries that sometimes are important collaterals in the intestinal circulation. A straight tube graft or an aortobiiliac bypass graft is used for the aortic reconstruction. A collagen-coated woven Dacron graft is recommended; these types of grafts are presealed with albumin and do not need preclotting. A tube graft is used if aorta is soft and not dilated at its bifurcation. If the dilation continues down into any of the common iliac arteries or if there are extensible calcifications in the bifurcation, a tube graft should not be used. If the iliac arteries are calcified or dilated extension of the graft limbs to the common femoral arteries may be necessary. This is combined with ligation of the common iliac arteries. The proximal anastomosis is usually sewn with nonresorbable monofilic 3-0 or 4-0 suture. When the graft is anastomosed to the iliac or femoral arteries a 5-0 suture is used.

After the reconstruction is complete, the anastomoses are checked for leakage and possible obstruction. Finally, the aneurysmal sac is wrapped around the graft and the dorsal peritoneum closed over it. Abdominal drains are never used because even significant postoperative bleeding cannot be drained. More about bleeding complications after aortic surgery can be found in Chapter 12 (page 149). The most common causes for postoperative bleeding are lumbar arteries not being secured during the procedure, anastomotic leakage, or veins that were not ligated but being temporarily contracted during the operation and later dilated.

Because of the increased risk of bleeding, systemic heparin should not be given to all patients with ruptured aneurysms. Those hemodynamically stable and with little operative bleeding should be given heparin IV. A recommendation is to use half the dose used for elective procedures. Local heparinization should be administered by infusing heparinized saline into the iliac arteries. Liberal use of Fogarty catheters to remove clots and emboli dislodged to the leg arteries from the thrombus during dissection is also advocated. If there is no backbleeding from either one of the common iliac arteries, thrombectomy is mandatory.

Antibiotic prophylaxis should be administered according to local protocols for operations involving synthetic vascular grafts. One suggestion is 2 g cloxacillin given at the start of the operation, with the dose repeated after 4 h in prolonged procedures. Besides general perioperative IV fluids, mannitol is recommended to maintain urinary output.

7.5.2.5 What to do While Waiting for Help

For surgeons without experience in AAA surgery it is generally a good idea to wait for a more experienced colleague if the patient is reasonably stable. While the surgeon is waiting for help the patient should be prepared up to the point of anesthesia induction. The surgeon scrubs and the patient is also scrubbed and draped while the anesthesiologist closely monitors the patient's vital functions and hemodynamics. If the patient's blood pressure drops and cannot be maintained at an acceptable level, the patient is anesthetized and laparotomy is initiated without experienced help. The goal is then to achieve control of the bleeding. Besides the previously described techniques to gain proximal control of the aorta, tamponade with lots of swabs and compression with the fist over the bleeding area is usually enough in this situation. These simple measures combined with IV fluids and inotropic drugs is often sufficient to stabilize the patient until help arrives.

7.5.2.6 Endovascular Treatment

In recent years more than 300 patients with ruptured AAA or incipient rupture have been treated with endovascular techniques. The results presented are observational studies and show that endovascular repair of rupture is feasible. A large percentage of the patients in these early series were not in severe shock and the mortality rate averaged around 10%. Furthermore, reduced postoperative morbidity rates compared with conventional open repair have been suggested.

One major benefit of endovascular treatment is the possibility of obtaining rapid proximal control by inserting an inflatable balloon from the groin or through the brachial artery that occludes aorta. This technique makes it possible to delay final treatment until the patient is stabilized. Another potential advantage may be that high-risk patients can also be treated. Particularly favorable is the possibility of using only local anesthesia and sedation for repair.

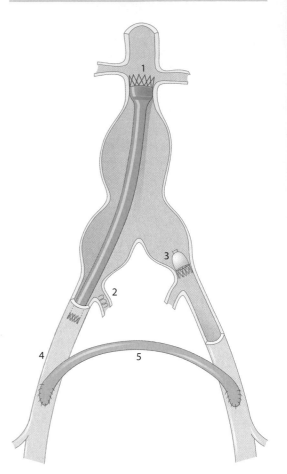

Fig. 7.6. One alternative way to treat a ruptured AAA with endovascular technique. A unilateral aortoiliac endovascular graft decompresses the aortic aneurysm. A coil in the right internal iliac artery and an occluder in the left common iliac artery eliminate pressure caused by backflow, the latter deployed to allow retrograde flow to the internal iliac artery from the groin. A femorofemoral bypass restores perfusion of the left leg

The problems related to endovascular repair include the availability and storage of suitable grafts as well as logistical problems getting the patients worked up rapidly. Pretreatment evaluation with CT angiography or digital subtraction arteriography is necessary to evaluate the possibility for endovascular repair and to plan the procedure. The number of different grafts needed to meet individual requirements is minimized if a unilateral aortoiliac tube graft is used in combination with an occluder of the contralateral iliac system and a femorofemoral crossover, as shown in Fig. 7.6.

The technique involves the following steps: The patient is prepped and draped as for an elective AAA procedure. The common femoral arteries are surgically exposed if a bifurcated graft is inserted or if unilateral aortoiliac tube grafts in combination with a femorofemoral crossover bypass are used. For tube grafts access of only one common femoral artery is enough. One of the femoral arteries is punctured and an introducer is put in place, often a size 7 to 9-French. A guide wire is inserted, an aortogram obtained, and landmarks, either radiolucent (placed preoperatively) or external (such as clamps), are used to assess the length of the AAA. After systemic heparinization, the sheath with the graft is introduced over the guide wire to a level just below the renal arteries. The sheath is then withdrawn somewhat to allow proximal release of the graft. After final adjustment of the proximal fixation level the system is secured by angioplasty. The distal end of the endoluminal graft is deployed in the common, external iliac, or common femoral artery with angioplasty of stents. Depending on the conditions a hand-sewn anastomosis is another option. An occluder of the common iliac is inserted from the contralateral femoral artery. If a bifurcated endoluminal graft is used, the contralateral graft limb is inserted through the same route. Finally, a completion angiogram is performed after withdrawal of the entire sheath.

A bifurcated aortobiiliac endoluminal prosthesis as a primary alternative in rupture is also growing in popularity. The procedure requires a compliant large-diameter balloon for aortic occlusion, 5 and 12-French introducers, Amplatz guide wires, high-resolution fluoroscopy, and an assortment of endoluminal aortic stent grafts with a body diameters ranging from 22 to 34 mm and limb diameters of 12 to 24 mm.

7.5.3 Management After Treatment

The patient is treated in the intensive care unit until circulatory, respiratory, and renal functions are stable. This usually takes at least a couple of days. The most common early postoperative complications are congestive heart failure, renal failure, and ischemic colitis. The patient, often with concomitant coronary heart disease, is exposed to severe stress during preoperative shock and aortic clamping and declamping. Deterioration of cardiac function with secondary hypotension that requires inotropic treatment is common. Renal function is also often impaired and occasionally the patient requires dialysis. Almost all patients have increased creatinine and blood urea nitrogen elevations after operation for ruptured AAA. These increases are also due to preoperative hypotension and the stress of the operation. If the patient develops renal insufficiency with low urinary output, dialysis should be considered at an early stage.

The greatest risk for developing ischemic colitis is in patients with a ruptured aneurysm and shock. The severity of ischemic colitis varies from only discharge of the mucosa to transmural necrosis. Registration of pH at the wall of the sigmoid with a tonometer can be used to determine the risk for developing ischemic colitis. This condition is further discussed in Chapter 12 on complications in vascular surgery (page 145).

7.6 Results and Outcome

The 30-day mortality after surgery for ruptured AAA averages from 30% to 50%, the variability depending on whether the patient developed shock and whether concomitant diseases were present. For patients without shock, it is 20–25%, which can be compared to 60–70% for those without. The long-term results and prognosis for patients who survive the initial postoperative period is good. Outcome is even better than for patients who have undergone elective aneurysm repair. The reason for this is probably selection – the sickest patients die of rupture, and the survivors who reach the hospital have fewer risk factors.

7.7 Unusual Types of Aortic Aneurysms

7.7.1 Inflammatory Aneurysm

An AAA can be symptomatic and cause pain without actual or imminent rupture. The most common cause for this pain is an inflammatory reaction in and around the wall – an inflammato-

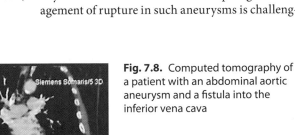

Fig. 7.7. Typical appearance on computed tomography of an inflammatory abdominal aortic aneurysm with its thick wall

7.7.2 Aortocaval Fistula

A special form of AAA rupture occurs when the bloodstream penetrates into the vena cava causing an aortocaval fistula (Fig. 7.8). The patient typically develops sudden cardiac failure and cyanosis of the lower extremities. The cardiac failure is due to the large shunt and the discoloration of the legs occurs because of venous stasis in combination with the heart failure. At physical examination the patient is positive for a bruit and a palpable aneurysm in the abdomen. Treatment for an aortocaval fistula is an emergency operation, but in most cases some time for preoperative preparation is available. The operation follows the strategy for other aneurysms as outlined previously and the fistula is usually closed by suture from inside the aneurysm while vena cava is controlled by manual compression proximally and distally.

7.7.3 Thoracoabdominal Aneurysm

A small number of aortic aneurysms engage the suprarenal or thoracoabdominal parts of the aorta including the orifices of the renal arteries, the superior mesenteric artery, and the celiac trunk. They originate in the thoracic part of the aorta or anywhere below the level of the diaphragm. Management of rupture in such aneurysms is challeng-

ry AAA. CT, which then shows a thickened aneurysm wall, verifies the presence of such a condition (Fig. 7.7). It could be presumed that the thick wall prevents rupture, but rupture of inflammatory AAAs is not uncommon. Because inflammatory AAAs often are painful, separating them from ruptured AAAs is a real diagnostic problem. Elevated erythrocyte sedimentation rate (ESR) or C-reactive protein (CRP) supports the diagnosis, but CT is the only way to exclude it.

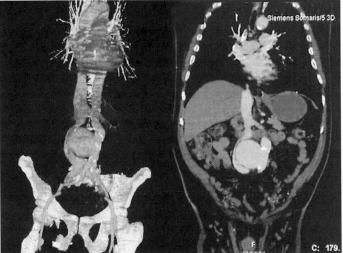

Fig. 7.8. Computed tomography of a patient with an abdominal aortic aneurysm and a fistula into the inferior vena cava

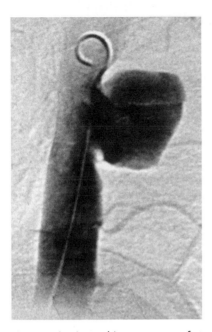

Fig. 7.9. Angiographic appearance of a typical mycotic aneurysm, with its saccular shape caused by local erosion of the aortic wall and subsequent leakage of blood into an aneurysmal sac consisting of a fibrous capsule (not a true vascular wall)

ing, and if its extension is known prior to the operation someone with experience should be contacted before surgery begins. If such an aneurysm is achieved during surgery for rupture, proximal control is sought by one of the techniques described previously. Endovascular repair is also an option that needs to be considered.

7.7.4 Mycotic Aneurysm

Another special type of AAA is caused by a local infection in an atherosclerotic and degenerated aortic wall, known as mycotic or septic aneurysm. Different from ordinary AAAs that are fusiform, mycotic aneurysms are usually saccular (Fig. 7.9). Patients with this type of AAA frequently have a medical history that includes fever and malaise. Elevated ESR, CRP, and other inflammatory parameters are also common. The most common bacteria found in mycotic aneurysms and in the patient's blood are of the Salmonella species. It is the infectious process in the wall that causes ero-

sion and subsequently rupture. Treatment is the same as for other AAAs with the addition of long-term antibiotics.

7.8 Ethical Considerations

Difficult and delicate ethical considerations often arise when managing patients with ruptured AAA. Accordingly, it has to be emphasized that the advice given above often needs to be modified in very old patients, patients with dementia, and patients with other serious medical conditions implying only a short expected survival time. On the other hand, patients who previously were determined not suitable for elective repair because of high risk should sometimes be considered for repair of a ruptured AAA. When rupture has already occurred the risk/benefit situation is completely different. The patient has little to lose by undergoing an emergency operation.

Rupture of an AAA often occurs in elderly patients and a complete medical history and information about their present quality of life is frequently missing when they are admitted. Because nonsurgical management is associated with 100% mortality, a policy of accepting every patient for surgical treatment is advocated in many hospitals. A certain selectivity, however, is often wise. It is obvious that a patient who had cardiac arrest in the ambulance and remains unconscious at admission, is anuric, and has ECG signs of myocardial ischemia is extremely unlikely to survive surgery. If the patient is 80 years old and also is known to have dementia, difficulties ambulating, and need for geriatric care, it is reasonable to avoid surgery and instead give the patient terminal care of high quality. Unfortunately, there are no reliable prognostic factors for treatment outcome for the individual patient, but many studies report relationships between presence of different risk factors and survival.

A common conclusion in the literature, however, is that age should never be considered as a contraindication to surgery. It is always the surgeon, the patient and relatives and their individual judgment that finally decide whether to operate or not. If one is in doubt, a good general rule is to be liberal with repair attempts. It is always possible, but difficult, to change such a strategy later during the course when more information is available. Accordingly, stopping the support of vital functions and taking the patient to the floor for palliation is a viable option. Some factors in the postoperative course – large bleedings and cardiac, renal, respiratory, and infectious complications – are considered to be associated with a worse prognosis and thus might indicate a suitable point at which to make such a decision.

■ Further Reading

Bengtsson H, Bergquist D. Ruptured abdominal aortic aneurysm: a population-based study. J Vasc Surg 1993; 18:74–80

Harris LM, Faggioli GL, Fiedler R et al. Ruptured abdominal aortic aneurysms: factors affecting mortality rates. J Vasc Surg 1991; 14:812–820

Johansson G, Swedenborg J. Ruptured abdominal aortic aneurysms: a study of incidence and mortality. Br J Surg 1986; 73:101–103

Johnston KW. Ruptured abdominal aortic aneurysms: six-year follow-up of a multicenter prospective study. J Vasc Surg 1994; 19:888–900

Ouriel K, Geary K, Green RM, et al. Factors determining survival after ruptured aortic aneurysm: the hospital, the surgeon, and the patient. J Vasc Surg 1990; 12:28–33

Ohki T, Veith FJ. Endovascular grafts and other image-guided catheter-based adjuncts to improve the treatment of ruptured aortoiliac aneurysms. Ann Surg 2000; 232(4):466–479

Aortic Dissection

8

CONTENTS

◼ 8.1 Summary

- ◼ Aortic dissection is one of the "great masqueraders," so always suspect this diagnosis in any acute painful illness with a pulse deficit.
- ◼ A practical classification in the emergency situation is type A, involving the ascending thoracic aorta and the arch and type B involving the aorta distal to the left subclavian artery.
- ◼ Treatment of type A dissection is always surgical.
- ◼ Treatment of type B dissection is medical in most cases and surgical if there is complicating organ ischemia or bleeding.
- ◼ Alert the attending thoracic or vascular surgeon on call early during management, especially in type A dissections.

◼ 8.2 Background

Dissection of the thoracic aorta represents a major clinical problem that is extremely demanding to manage even for experienced surgeons. Once it is diagnosed this condition is usually managed by an experienced specialist in thoracic or vascular surgery. The responsibility for the diagnosis and its primary management, however, mostly belongs to the surgical or medical emergency physicians.

◼ 8.2.1 Magnitude of the Problem

The true prevalence and incidence of aortic dissection are unknown, but it has been reported to have an annual occurrence of 5–10 cases per million and to affect between 10,000 and 25,000 patients annually in the United States. Autopsy studies in the United States and Denmark report dissections in 0.2–0.8% and 0.2% of cases, respectively. An age-adjusted mortality rate from aortic dissections of 0.5–2.7% per 100,000 inhabitants was calculated from 1950 to 1981. The overall incidence of aortic dissections consequently is in the same range or possibly up to two to three times greater than that for ruptured abdominal aortic aneurysm. It is two to five times more common in men than in women, and maximum occurrence is in the 5th decade of life. Still, in our era of modern diagnostic methods, a majority of patients probably die with this disease undetected. Aortic dissection is a dramatic and dangerous condition with a very high mortality: 20–50% of patients die within the first 24–48 h, and up to 75% within the first 2 weeks. It is considered as one of the "great masqueraders," with a wide range of presenting symptoms. Because the diagnosis is difficult, awareness of aortic dissection in the differential diagnosis is essential, as is rapid and correct management.

8.2.2 Classification and Definition

Aortic dissection is characterized by two or more communicating flow channels originating from a proximal intimal tear, with propagation of the bloodstream within the medial layer. It should be distinguished from an intramural hematoma, which is a hemorrhage into the medial layer of the aortic wall without an intimal tear. Intramural hematomas have a natural history similar to aortic dissection and are treated similarly.

The most useful classification of aortic dissections in the acute situation is the one proposed by Daily (Stanford classification), as shown in Fig. 8.1.

Other classic classifications are by DeBakey and Crawford (thoracoabdominal aneurysms and chronic dissections). The information in this chapter is based on the Stanford classification because it simplifies the acute management. A type-A dissection always involves the ascending aorta, regardless of the distal extension. A type-B dissection does not involve the ascending aorta. There is consensus in the literature that an aortic dissection is considered acute if the onset of symptoms occurred

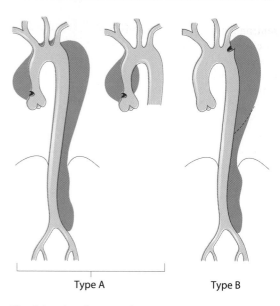

Type A   Type B

Fig. 8.1. Classification of aortic dissection in types A and B, according to Daily (Stanford)

within 14 days of presentation, and chronic if more than 14 days have elapsed.

NOTE
The most practical classification in the emergency situation is
– **Type A: involving the ascending thoracic aorta and the arch**
– **Type B: involving the aorta distal to the left subclavian artery**

8.2.3 Etiology

Aortic dissection is usually related to some kind of degenerative changes in the aortic wall, in particular the media. Even if a dissection primarily starts with a tear in the intima, its propagation within the media varies considerably from almost none to rapid progression along the entire length of the aorta. The variation is related to the condition of the medial layer. Some congenital connective tissue defects are known to cause such degeneration, including Marfan's syndrome, Turner syndrome, and Ehlers–Danlos' syndrome. Cystic media necrosis is another predisposing condition. The role of arteriosclerosis is often discussed. It is present in older patients with hypertension presenting with dissection and might constitute a rare mechanism by penetration of atherosclerotic ulcers extending through the intima into the media. This is, however, mostly considered coincidental rather than causative, and some authors even argue that atherosclerotic changes within the aortic wall might be a barrier to the extension of a dissection.

Arterial hypertension is the most important predisposing factor. It is noteworthy that the sudden extreme hypertension associated with severe physical exercise may cause aortic dissection in younger persons. Also, pregnancy with its hyper-circulation and hormonal changes affecting connective tissue, is a certain risk factor particularly during the last trimester and during labor. Fortunately, aortic dissections in women are rare, but 50% of dissections occurring in women younger than 40 years old do occur during pregnancy.

Iatrogenic injuries during coronary diagnostic and therapeutic procedures with catheter manipulations can also cause aortic dissection. Blunt chest trauma in otherwise healthy persons may cause aortic dissection, but such dissections are usually very limited due to the minimal degeneration in these structurally normal aortas.

NOTE

A degenerative process causing weakening of the aortic wall in combination with hypertension is the most important etiologic factor.

■ 8.2.4 Pathophysiology

Type A dissection, constituting 60–70% of all aortic dissections, is mostly seen in younger patients with some elastic and connective tissue abnormality. It characteristically starts with a primary intimal tear just distal to the sinotubular ridge in the ascending aorta. This location is in the vicinity of the cephalad extension of the aortic valve commissures. The tear is commonly transverse and has a length corresponding to 50–60% of the aortic circumference. The dissection process starts in the intimal tear and its extension and direction vary, as does the speed with which it propagates.

Typically, a type A dissection affects the right lateral wall of the greater curvature of the ascending aorta. The dissection is usually directed antegradely, but retrograde extension is also relatively common. A primary entry in the ascending aorta is associated with a great risk for bleeding into the pericardium, causing cardiac tamponade.

Type B dissection usually starts with a primary intimal tear in the descending thoracic aorta just distal to the origin of left subclavian artery. This type constitutes approximately 25% of all aortic dissections. A patient with a type-B dissection is typically older, in the 6th–7th decade of life, and has thoracic aortic degeneration and hypertension.

Other possible but less common sites of the primary tear are the aortic arch, occurring in approximately 10% of cases, and the abdominal aorta, occurring in only 2%. As already mentioned, the dissection in the aortic media can travel in a retrograde as well as an antegrade direction, causing two flow channels with a false and a true lumen. Secondary tears and reentries usually occur distally, allowing flow from the false into the true lumen.

Rupture is the most common cause of death in patients with aortic dissection and is mostly located near the site of the primary intimal tear. Consequently, a type-A dissection usually ruptures into the pericardial sac, causing cardiac tamponade, or an aortic arch rupture that bleeds into the mediastinum. In addition, the close relation to the aortic valve commisures can result in acute valve regurgitation due to prolapse of the commissural attachments. Dissection into the aortic root may also involve the coronary arteries, leading to myocardial ischemia or infarction. A type-B descending aortic dissection typically ruptures into the left pleural cavity, and less frequently into the right.

As the dissection extends along the aorta it will subsequently engage major important cerebral and visceral branches, possibly resulting in threatening end-organ ischemia. The mechanisms behind this are compression of the true lumen by the false lumen or shearing of the branch by the dissection process. A third possibility is disruption of an important dissection membrane, causing an intimal flap covering the orifice of a branch. Such peripheral vascular complications occur in 25–30% of patients with aortic dissection and can critically affect cerebral, renal, visceral, and lower

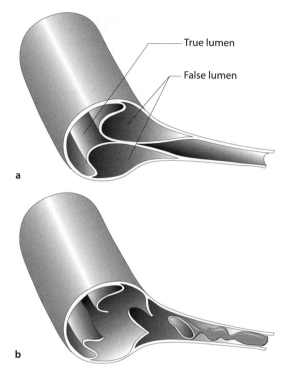

Fig. 8.2. Mechanisms of branch occlusion and organ malperfusion in aortic dissection. **a** False lumen expansion causes compression of a side branch. **b** The orifice of a side branch is disrupted by dissection, and its inner layers are impacted distally

extremity perfusion. Because the dissection in the descending aorta mainly engages its left perimeter, the left renal and left iliac arteries are at higher risk than the right ones.

NOTE

> Peripheral vascular complications occur in 25–30% of cases of dissection of the aorta.

8.3 Clinical Presentation

8.3.1 Signs and Symptoms

Acute aortic dissection patients can display a variety of symptoms, and affected individuals can develop symptoms mimicking those of almost any other acute medical or surgical condition. Aortic dissection must be considered in patients presenting with symptoms indicating acute arterial occlusion and an acute illness that seems to involve unrelated organ systems.

8.3.2 Medical History

The most dominant symptom is severe pain, which is migrating or nonmigrating and experienced by more than 90% of patients. When analyzing the pain its typical characteristics are evaluated; if it is: sudden, severe, new, ripping or tearing, and constant. The pain is typically related to the location of the dissection and its propagation distally into different aortic segments. In proximal dissection, the most common pain location is the anterior chest. The pain frequently radiates into the neck and jaws and can be associated with swallowing difficulties. As the dissection propagates distally, the pain migrates to an interscapular location followed by pain in the midback, lumbar, and groin regions (Fig. 8.3).

Abdominal pain might be severe in patients suffering from visceral or renal ischemia. As previously mentioned, the left renal artery is more likely to be compromised, which may explain why severe left flank pain mimicking ureteral colic is often included in the reported history. One should always include questions about hypertension, cardiac disease, peripheral vascular disease, connective tissue abnormalities (such as Marfan's, Turner, and Ehlers–Danlos' syndromes), cystic media ne-

Table 8.1. Differential diagnoses in aortic dissection

Possible differential diagnoses
Coronary ischemia
Myocardial infarction
Aortic regurgitation without dissection
Aortic aneurysm with dissection
Musculoskeletal pain
Mediastinal tumors or cysts
Pericarditis
Gall bladder disease
Pulmonary embolism
Stroke
Visceral or lower extremity ischemia without dissection

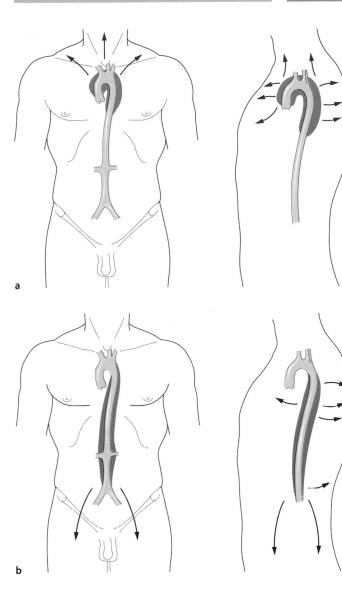

Fig. 8.3. a Radiation of pain in type A dissection. The pain is usually referred to the neck, anterior chest, and interscapular area. **b** Radiation of pain in type B dissection. Pain is primarily interscapular, but with distal progression of dissection, pain is often referred to the lower back and groin

a

b

crosis, diagnostic or therapeutic catheter manipulations, or intense exercise.

Secondary effects of aortic dissection with organ malperfusion necessitate a thorough and complete history to include previous, present, and undulating symptoms of the following:

- Cerebral ischemia: stroke, loss of consciousness, focal neurological symptoms
- Spinal ischemia: paraplegia or parapareses
- Renal ischemia: flank pain, hematuria, diminished urinary output

- Visceral ischemia: severe abdominal pain (for further details of typical symptoms, see Chapter 6, p. 67)
- Lower-extremity ischemia: loss of pulse, loss of sensory or/and motor function, severe pain and coldness (see Chapter 10, p. 122)
- Cardiac malperfusion: angina pectoris or symptoms of acute congestive heart failure

Possible differential diagnoses are listed in Table 8.1.

NOTE

Be aware of aortic dissection as an important differential diagnosis in any acute case presenting with sudden painful illness, in particular if it is associated with symptoms or signs of organ ischemia.

■ 8.3.3 Physical Examination

Complete and repeated physical examinations are of paramount importance in diagnosing and managing patients with suspected or verified acute aortic dissection since this condition can affect so many different organ systems and has a dynamic course.

The typical patient presents with paradoxical physical findings. He or she is frequently pale, restless, and in preshock or shock, and has an appearance indicating poor peripheral perfusion but with a paradoxically high blood pressure. Eighty percent of the patients have arterial hypertension at admission. The high blood pressure is secondary to underlying essential hypertension, elevated catecholamine levels due to severe pain, or occlusion of the renal arteries or even the thoracic or abdominal aorta.

Twenty percent of the patients have a low blood pressure instead. This is usually secondary to cardiac tamponade or rupture, or to acute congestive heart failure secondary to acute aortic insufficiency. Another possible explanation is pseudo-hypotension secondary to mechanical obstruction from the dissection of one or both subclavian arteries.

Auscultation of the chest is of vital importance. A cardiac murmur indicates aortic regurgitation. The first heart sound is diminished or absent due to elevated end diastolic ventricular pressure. There might be an S3 gallop rhythm. A continuous murmur usually indicates rupture into the right atrium. A pericardial friction rub indicates leakage into the pericardial sac. Auscultation of the lungs might reveal signs of pulmonary edema. Loss of alveolar breath sounds can be found after leakage or rupture into one or both of the pleural cavities. Jugular venous distension is also a common finding.

A complete and repeated neurological examination is mandatory. Horner's syndrome, loss of consciousness, loss of sensory or motor function, paraparesis, paralysis, or paraplegia might be present. Acute cerebral vascular occlusion is for obvious anatomic reasons, more common in proximal dissection, but fortunately neurological deficits occur in only about 20% of those patients.

Lower extremity paralysis in the examination is caused by shearing off or compression of major arteries feeding the spinal cord (intercostal-T8–L1). Another possible explanation is occlusion of the thoracic or abdominal aorta, causing ischemia of the lower body including peripheral nerves. The clinical distinction is important because spinal cord ischemia has a poor prognosis, while a peripheral nerve ischemia has a better prognosis if treated. This distinction can be made by examining peripheral pulses. The latter condition is usually combined with loss of pulses in the groins and distally in the affected lower extremities.

Repeated examination of peripheral pulses as well as blood pressures in the arms and ankles are important indicators of the extension of a dissection and its consequences of organ malperfusion. Repeated examinations are important in order to follow the development. A peripheral pulse may disappear, or a pulse deficit may be dynamic and resolve spontaneously, which is reported to occur in one-third of the patients. Such a dynamic course is probably related to redirection of flow from the false into the true lumen after spontaneous fenestration of the aortic septum known as the reentry phenomenon.

A new pulse deficit is found in approximately 60% of the patients.

■ 8.4 Diagnostics

An electrocardiogram (ECG) should be obtained in the emergency department. Low voltage might indicate pericardial tamponade, and ST–T wave changes could indicate myocardial ischemia.

The following blood tests should be ordered: complete blood cell count, arterial blood gases, protrombin and thromboplastin times, serum electrolytes, creatinine, blood urea nitrogen, liver enzymes and lactate.

As with the physical examination, repeated blood tests according to the patient's clinical course might be of great diagnostic value during the acute stage of the disease. Mild anemia is common, while severe anemia indicates rupture and bleeding. Hemolysis with elevated bilirubin or lactic acid concentrations can also be found. A leukocytosis with a count of 10,000–15,000 is common. Blood gases might reveal a metabolic acidosis due to anaerobic metabolism in ischemic tissue. Urinary tests showing hematuria indicates renal involvement.

A plain chest x-ray in standard anteroposterior and lateral projections is rarely diagnostic, but the following findings indicates the presence of aortic dissection:

- Abnormal shadow adjacent to the descending thoracic aorta
- Deformity of the aortic knob
- Density adjacent to the brachiocephalic trunk
- Enlarged cardiac shadow
- Displaced esophagus, trachea, or bronchus
- Abnormal mediastinum
- Irregular aortic contour
- Loss of sharpness of the aortic shadow
- Pleural effusion
- Expanded aortic diameter

Helical CT is accurate for determining the presence of an aortic dissection and provides information for classification. The identification of an intimal tear is, however, difficult and motion artifacts of the ascending aorta are sometimes misinterpreted as dissection. MRI is highly accurate and gives valuable information about the pathoanatomy. Unfortunately it cannot be performed in hemodynamically unstable patients who are on ventilator support.

TEE (Transesophageal echocardiography) is often considered as one of the most valuable diagnostic tools, making it possible to determine the type and extent of the aortic dissection, especially distally. It has limitations in visualization of the distal ascending aorta and the arch. TTE (Transthoracic echocardiography) is, on the other hand, superior for evaluating involvement of the proximal part of the descending aorta in the dissection. Together, TEE and TTE yield a sensitivity and specificity approaching 100% for diagnosing dissection and are thus probably the best – but unfortunately often not available – diagnostic modalities.

Aortography is the old gold standard and is highly accurate in diagnosing aortic dissection, but it can fail to recognize a thrombosed false lumen. It also provides better information than CT or MRI about the condition and involvement of the aortic branches. Furthermore, aortography can be combined with therapeutic endovascular management. However, the modern CT scanners with up to 64 detectors can produce extremely detailed images and, when available, should be the first imaging study after the chest x-ray.

8.5 Management

8.5.1 Treatment in the Emergency Department

As soon as aortic dissection is clinically suspected, aggressive medical treatment must be started immediately. The goals are to (1) stabilize dissection, (2) prevent rupture, and (3) prevent organ ischemia.

These goals can be achieved by diminishing the stress on the aortic wall. Consequently, the therapeutic cornerstone is to reduce blood pressure in order to minimize the force of the left ventricular ejection (dP/dT). The reduction in blood pressure must, however, be balanced against what is needed for adequate cerebral, coronary, renal, and visceral perfusion. A useful guideline is that the systolic arterial blood pressure should be kept around 100–110 mmHg and mean arterial pressure between 60 and 75 mmHg, provided that urinary output and neurology are unaffected.

In the emergency department the following measures can be employed:

1. Insert one or two large-bore intravenous (IV) lines for administering antihypertensive drugs and fluids.
2. Obtain an ECG.
3. Order blood tests as stated above.
4. Obtain a plain chest x-ray.
5. Administer oxygen by mask
6. Consider injection of a strong analgesic IV, such as morphine 5–10-mg.
7. Insert an arterial catheter for blood pressure monitoring.

8. Start administration of a beta-blocker as described below.

The recommended agents for medical management of acute aortic dissection are direct vasodilators, beta-blockers, nitroglycerin and calcium channel blockers if beta blockers cannot be used.

Beta-blockers orally are recommended for all patients. Contraindications for beta-blockers are heart failure, bradyarrhythmias, atrioventricular blocks, and bronchospastic disease.

Suggested emergency medical treatment (local variations in drug choices are of course common) is as follows:

Start propranolol treatment, 1 mg IV, every 3–5 min until achieving a systolic blood pressure around 100 mmHg and a heart rate of 60–80 beats/min (maximum dose, up to 0.15 mg/kg). Continue thereafter with 2–6 mg IV every 4–6 h. In patients with severe hypertension an IV infusion of nitroglycerin is started and the dose titrated after blood pressure and heart rate.

NOTE

The main objective of the medical treatment is to lower the blood pressure to a level of 100–110 mmHg. It is mandatory to check the patient for the development of new complications of the dissection during medical treatment.

8.5.2 Emergency Surgery

Emergency surgery should be considered in type A dissections involving the intrapericardial ascending aorta and the aortic arch. A distal type B dissection with retrograde dissection involving the aortic arch is also a case for acute operation. A double aortic lumen in the pericardial portion of the ascending aorta is an absolute indication for emergency operation. Depending on the patient's general condition prior to the dissection there are, as usual, exceptions from these basic rules. Contraindications include very advanced age and severe debilitating or terminal illnesses.

Surgical repair of the condition requires thoracic surgical expertise and includes replacing the ascending aorta and resecting the primary intimal tear. The operation involves cardiopulmonary by

pass. In type A dissection with persistent organ ischemia despite open surgical repair and replacement of the ascending aorta, endovascular treatment of the rest of the dissection is often a successful complement.

8.5.3 Type B dissection

The management of acute distal aortic dissection is initially always medical because this results in lower morbidity and mortality than emergent surgical repair. Consequently, the continued regimen for these patients follows the previously given recommendations regarding beta blockade and vasodilators started in the emergency department.

The medical treatment must be combined with careful observation for complications. Surgical or endovascular intervention should be considered for the following situations:

- Aortic rupture
- Increasing periaortic or intrapleural fluid (suggesting aneurysmal leakage)
- Rapidly expanding aortic diameter
- Uncontrolled hypertension
- Persistent pain despite adequate medical therapy
- Organ malperfusion – ischemia of brain, spinal cord, abdominal viscera, or limbs

The goal of surgical repair in a type B dissection is, as with all other treatment options, to prevent rupture and restore visceral and limb perfusion. Because a common site of rupture is associated with the site of primary dissection, at least the upper half of the descending thoracic aorta needs to be replaced in most cases. Graft replacement in the acute setting should be limited and replacement of the entire thoracic aorta avoided if possible. An abdominal fenestration procedure is sometimes necessary to restore flow to the lower extremities. Extraanatomical by pass is another possible way to reestablish flow to the legs.

8.5.4 Endovascular Treatment

In patients with peripheral vascular complications due to extension of the dissection into a branch, causing compression and obstruction of its true

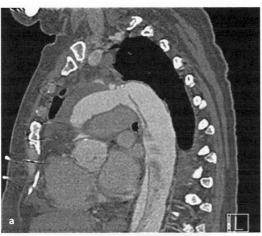

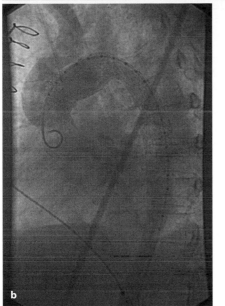

Fig. 8.4. a Computed tomography showing a type B dissection and its entry in the first part of the descending aorta in a patient with a previous reconstruction of the arch and the brachiocephalic trunk after a type A dissection. The true anterior aortic lumen is severely compressed causing obstruction of the main visceral branches and leading to visceral ischemia. **b** Flow into the true aortic lumen and all branches is restored after deploying a covered stent over the entry site in the descending aorta

lumen, as well as in patients with central aortic true lumen collapse, the endovascular option should be considered. Provided, of course, that the institution has technically skilled physicians, the necessary equipment and back-up support. It is possible to create a fenestration through the intimal flap from the false into the true lumen with endovascular techniques. As shown in Fig. 8.2 a, stenting of the entry site to occlude flow into the false lumen will probably be successful in restoring flow into a branch with its orifice obstructed by the false lumen and the dissection membrane. If there is an avulsion of the intima of that branch as in Fig. 8.2 b, this is not an option.

Endovascular management is developing as an attractive alternative to surgical repair. Patients with an acute type B dissection who are not good candidates for surgery can be considered for endovascular management. Stenting has also been reported to give successful results in aortic collapse with severe ischemia of the lower part of the body.

An endovascular approach can also be used as the initial treatment by performing aortic fenestration and stenting. Most centers prefer to delay either surgical or endovascular repair until after the patient has recovered from the acute phase of malperfusion, whereas others advocate early prophylactic stenting and coverage of the intimal tear to occlude the false lumen and prevent further dissection (Fig. 8.4).

8.6 Results and Outcome

A recent article from 12 international centers covering 464 patients with aortic dissection reported, in-hospital mortality rates for type-A dissections treated surgically of 28%, and medically of 58%. The corresponding figures for type B were 31% and 10%, respectively.

Successful closure of the intimal tear with endovascular stent grafts and subsequent thrombosis of the false lumen is reported in up to 75% of patients. Branch occlusions with ischemic symptoms were relieved in 75–95% of the cases. Survival after 30 days was 75–85 %, and long-term results are good, with <1% related deaths and verified thrombosis of the false lumen in 100% of the survivors. No thromboembolic complications occured. In general, survival is lower for patients with paraplegia or visceral or renal ischemia. In cases with type B dissections and indications for surgical intervention, the results of endovascular intervention seem more favorable compared with conventional surgical repair, but the number of reported cases from any single center is still low. In all cases, long-term follow-up regarding development of aneurysms and continued antihypertensive medication is essential.

■ Further Reading

Cambria RP, Brewster DC, Gertler, et al. Vascular complications associated with spontaneous aortic dissection. J Vasc Surg 1988; 7:199–209

Cigarroa JE, Isselbacher EM, DeSanctis RW, et al. Diagnostic imaging in the evaluation of suspected aortic dissections: Old standards and new directions. N Engl J Med 1993; 328:35–43

Daily PO, Trueblood HW, Stinson EB, et al. Management of acute aortic dissections. Ann Thorac Surg 1970; 10:237

De Bakey ME, McCollum CH, Crawford ES, et al. Dissection and dissecting aneurysms of the aorta: twenty year follow up of five hundred twenty-seven patients treated surgically. Surgery 1982; 92:1118

Hagan PG, Nienaber CA, Isselbacher EM, et al. The International Registry of Acute Aortic Dissection – new insights into an old disease. JAMA 2000; 283(7):897903

Lilienfeld DE, Gundersson PD, Sprafka JM, et al. Epidemiology of aortic aneurysms. Mortality trends in the United States, 1951–1981. Arteriosclerosis 1987; 7:637

Slonim SM, Miller DC, Mitchell RS, et al. Percutaneous Balloon fenestration and stenting for life threatening ischemic complications in patients with acute aortic dissection. J Thorac Cardiovasc Surg 1999; 117(6):1118–1126

Williams DM, Lee DY, Hamilton BH, et al. The dissected aorta: Percutaneous treatment of ischemic complications principles and results. J Vasc Interv Radiol 1997; 8:605-625

Vascular Injuries in the Leg

9

CONTENTS

■ 9.1 Summary

- Major bleeding is controlled by manual compression.
- Vascular injuries should always be suspected in extremities with fractures.
- Most vascular injuries are revealed by careful and repeated clinical examination.
- Obtain proximal control before exploring a wound in a patient with a history of substantial bleeding.

■ 9.2 Background

■ 9.2.1 Background

Vascular trauma to extremity vessels is caused by violent behavior or accidents. Because of the rise in the number of endovascular procedures, iatrogenic injuries have also become an increasing part of vascular trauma. Vascular injuries may cause life-threatening major bleeding, but distal ischemia is more common. Ischemia occurs after both blunt and penetrating trauma. The vascular injury is often one of many injuries in multiply traumatized patients that make the recognition of signs of vascular injury – which can be blurred by more apparent problems – and the diagnosis difficult. Table 9.1 lists common locations of combined orthopedic and vascular injury. Multiple injuries also bring problems regarding priority.

Table 9.1. Most common locations for combined orthopedic and vascular injury

Orthopedic injury	Vascular injury
Femoral shaft fracture	Superficial femoral artery
Knee dislocation	Popliteal artery
Fractured clavicle	Subclavian artery
Shoulder dislocation	Axillary artery
Supracondylar fracture of the humerus Elbow dislocation	Brachial artery

9.2.2 Magnitude of the Problem

Data on the true incidence of vascular injuries to the legs is hard to gather. The incidence of vascular trauma varies among countries and also between rural and urban areas. It is usually higher where gunshot wounds are common. There is an equal share of blunt and penetrating injury in most studies from Europe, whereas penetrating injury is slightly more common in the United States. Approximately 75% of all vascular injuries are localized to the extremities and more than 50% to the legs. The true incidence of iatrogenic trauma is unknown.

9.2.3 Etiology and Pathophysiology

9.2.3.1 Penetrating Injury

Penetrating vascular injury is caused by stab and cutting injuries, gunshots, and fractures, the latter when sharp bone fragments penetrate the vascular wall. Gunshots cause major bleeding by direct artery trauma, while high-velocity bullets create a cavitation effect with massive soft tissue destruction and secondary arterial damage. In fact, after all types of penetrating trauma both bleeding and indirect blunt arterial injury with ischemia may occur. Bleeding is more often exsanguinating after sharp injury and partial vessel transection. Complete avulsion, especially when caused by blunt trauma, makes the vessel more prone to retraction, spasm, and thrombosis. This diminishes the risk for major bleeding. Iatrogenic injuries can be caused by catheterization and during surgical dissection.

NOTE
Penetrating injuries can cause both major bleeding and ischemia.

9.2.3.2 Blunt Injury

Blunt vascular injuries are usually caused by motor vehicle and other accidents. The consequences are thrombosis and ischemia distal to the injured vessel. The media and the intimal layers of the vessel wall are easily separated, and subsequent dissection by the bloodstream between the layers may lead to lumen obstruction. Blunt injuries also induce thrombosis. This type of vessel injury is particularly common when the artery is hyperextended as in knee joint luxations and upper arm fractures. Contusion of the vessel may also cause bleeding in the vessel wall. Thrombosis and ischemia by this mechanism can occur several hours after the traumatic situation. Narrowing of the arterial lumen following blunt trauma is rarely caused by spasm and it can be disregarded as etiology.

9.2.3.3 Pathophysiology

The main pathophysiological issue after vascular injuries to the extremities is ischemia. The process is identical to what happens during acute leg ischemia due to embolization (see Chapter 10, p. 120). Irreversible damage to the distal parts of the legs is not infrequent and the diagnosis is more difficult to determine than for other types of leg ischemia. The reason is the multiple manifestations of the trauma. It must be kept in mind that the time limit for acute leg ischemia – 4–6 h before permanent changes occur – is also valid for trauma.

NOTE
Irreversible tissue damage may occur if more than 6 h passes before blood flow to the leg is restored.

A vascular injury missed during the initial examination may develop into a pseudoaneurysm or an arteriovenous fistula. A pseudoaneurysm is a hematoma with persistent blood flow within it that may enlarge over time and cause local symptoms and sometimes even rupture. When both an artery and an adjacent vein are injured simultaneously an arteriovenous fistula may develop. These can become quite large with time and even cause cardiac failure due to increased cardiac output.

9.3 Clinical Presentation

9.3.1 Medical History

Most patients with major vascular injury present with any or several of the "hard signs" of vessel injury (Table 9.2) and the diagnosis is obvious. Penetrating injury patients who arrive in the emergency department without active hemorrhage are usually not in shock because the bleeding was controlled at the trauma scene. Shock in patients with penetrating injury usually means that the bleeding is ongoing. Still, information about the trauma mechanism is often needed to estimate the likelihood for vessel injury and to facilitate the management process.

Besides interviewing the patient, additional background information may be available from medical personnel and accompanying persons. The few minutes required to establish a picture of the trauma situation are usually worthwhile. For example, a history of a large amount of bright red pulsating bleeding after penetrating trauma suggests a severe arterial injury. Venous bleedings are often described as a steady flow of dark red blood. In high-impact accidents the risk for a severe vascular injury is increased.

Besides being helpful when assessing the risk for a major injury estimation of the blood loss is also important for later volume replacement.

Knowledge of the exact time when the injury happened is helpful for determining the available time before irreversible damage occurs from ischemia. The duration of ischemia also influences the management priority in multitrauma patients, and the time elapsed affects the presentation of the ischemic symptoms. For example, an initial severe

Table 9.2. Signs of vascular injury

Hard signs	Soft signs
Active hemorrhage	History of significant bleeding
Hematoma (large, pulsating, expanding)	Small hematoma
Distal ischemia ("six Ps")	Adjacent nerve injury
Bruit	Proximity of wound to vessel location Unexplained shock

pain may vanish with time as a consequence of ischemic nerve damage. Even a major internal hemorrhage may be present without being clinically obvious after a very recent injury.

Information about complicating diseases and medication is also helpful. For instance, beta-blockers may abolish the tachycardia in hypovolemia.

9.3.2 Clinical Signs and Symptoms

The physical examination is performed after the primary and secondary surveys of a multitrauma patient and should focus on identifying major vessel injury. The examination should be thorough, especially regarding signs of distal ischemia. It should include examination and auscultation of the injured area, palpation of pulses in both legs, and assessment of skin temperature, motor function, and sensibility. The presence of one or more of the classic hard signs of vascular injury listed in Table 9.2 suggests that a major vessel is damaged and that immediate repair is warranted. Findings of "soft" signs should bring the examiner's attention to the fact that a major vessel may be injured but that the definite diagnosis requires additional work-up. As noted in Table 9.2, the hard sign of distal ischemia as suggested by the "six Ps" (see Chapter 10, p. 121) suggests vascular injury.

NOTE
Measurement of ankle pressure should always be included in the examination.

The principles of the vascular examination suggested for acute leg ischemia are also valid for vascular injuries, but certain details need to be emphasized. Vascular trauma in the legs usually strikes young persons, so it should be assumed that the patient had a normal vascular status before the injury. A palpable pulse does not exclude vascular injury; 25% of patients with arterial injuries that require surgical treatment have a palpable pulse initially. This is due to propagation of the pulse wave through soft thrombus. Pulses may be palpated initially in spite of an intimal flap or minor vessel wall narrowing and can later cause thrombosis and occlude the vessel. Ankle pressure measurements and calculation of the ankle brachial index (ABI) should therefore supplement palpation of pulses. If the ABI is ≤0.9, arterial injuries should be suspected.

Findings in the physical examination of a patient in shock are particularly difficult to interpret. In several aspects findings of distal ischemia caused by vascular injury are similar to vasoconstriction of the skin vessels in the foot. Differences in pallor, the presence of pulses, and skin temperature between the injured and uninjured leg therefore should be interpreted as the possible presence of vascular injury. Ankle pressure measurements are also valuable during such circumstances.

It is important to remember to listen for bruits and thrills over the wounded area to reveal a possible arteriovenous fistula.

■ 9.4 Diagnostics

Recommendations for management of suspected vascular injuries in the leg have evolved from mandatory exploration of all suspected injuries (a common practice during past wars), to routine angiography for most patients, to a more selective approach today. Regarding exploration and subsequent angiography, it was found that negative explorations and arteriograms were obtained in over 80% of the patients. The associated risk for complications and morbidity after these invasive procedures is the rationale for a more selective approach. Rapid transportation, clinical examination, ankle pressure measurements, careful monitoring, and duplex examination leave angiography for some of the patients and urgent exploration for a few.

■ 9.4.1 Angiography

Angiography is unnecessary when a vascular injury is obvious after the examination. The two most common indications for excluding vascular injury are (1) when there are no hard signs at the examination, and (2) when clinical findings are imprecise but the ABI is <0.9.

Angiography is more often indicated after blunt trauma than penetrating. The reason for this is the more difficult clinical examination because of the more extensive soft tissue and nerve damage after

blunt trauma. It may occasionally be helpful to perform angiography even when injury is evident in order to exactly locate the injured vessel. An option is to perform it intraoperatively. The technique is described in Chapter 10, p. 128. Contralateral puncture is important when the injury is close to the groin.

The purpose of the arteriography is to identify and locate lesions such as occlusions, narrowing, and intimal flaps. Contrast leakage outside the vessel can be visualized, and it also serves to provide a road map before surgery. It has, however, been argued that it is unnecessary to search for minimal lesions; some studies have shown that it is safe and effective to manage such lesions nonoperatively. On the other hand, angiography may be the first step in the final treatment of such small lesions by stenting.

When the injury is caused by a shotgun blast, angiography should always be performed because multiple vascular injuries are common. It is then indicated regardless of the clinical signs and symptoms. The risk for complications after angiography is very low, but the risk of complications is higher when the punctured artery is small. Children therefore have a rather high rate of complications. A contributing factor is that their very vasoactive arteries are prone to temporary spasm. Overall, as described above, the risk for complications after angiography does not warrant avoiding it when indicated.

Occasionally it is worthwhile to order venography. It may be indicated in patients not subjected to exploration because arterial injury was ruled out but in whom a major venous injury is suspected. As an example, 5–10% of all popliteal venous injuries are reported to occur without arterial damage.

■ 9.4.2 Duplex Ultrasound

Despite the usefulness of duplex scanning in general for vascular diagnosis, it has not been universally accepted for diagnosis of vascular trauma despite the fact that it is noninvasive. It is operator dependent and vessels may be difficult to assess in multiply injured patients, legs with skeletal deformities, large hematomas, and through splints and dressings. In some hospitals with expertise in duplex assessment and round-the-clock access to skilled examiners, duplex has replaced angiography to a large extent. The indications proposed are then the same as for angiography.

Duplex is also the method of choice for diagnosis of most of the late consequences of vascular injuries to the legs – arteriovenous fistulas, pseudoaneurysms, and hematomas.

9.5 Management and Treatment

9.5.1 Management Before Treatment

9.5.1.2 Severe Vessel Injury

Major external bleeding not adequately stopped when the patient arrives to the emergency department should immediately be controlled with digital pressure or bandages. No other measures to control bleeding are taken in the emergency department and attempts to clamp vessels are saved for the operating room.

The patient is surveyed according to the trauma principles used in the hospital. For most patients without obvious vascular injuries to the leg vessels, more careful vascular assessment takes place after the secondary survey. If the vascular injury is one of many in a multitrauma patient, general trauma principles for trauma care are applied. Treatment of the vascular problem is then initiated as soon as possible when the patient's condition allows it.

Patients with hard signs of vascular injury but without other problems should be transferred immediately to the operating room. Before transfer the following can be done:

1. Give the patient oxygen.
2. Initiate monitoring of vital signs (heart rate, blood pressure, respirations, SpO_2).
3. Place at least one large-bore intravenous (IV) line.
4. Start infusion of fluids. Dextran preceded by 20 ml Promiten is advised especially if the patient has distal ischemia.
5. Draw blood for hemoglobin and hematocrit, prothrombin time, partial thromboplastin time, complete blood count, creatinine, sodium, and potassium as well as a sample for blood type and cross-match.
6. Obtain informed consent.
7. Consider administering antibiotics and tetanus prophylaxis.
8. Consider administering analgesics (5–10 mg opiate IV).

9.5.1.2 Less Severe Injuries

ABI must be measured when vascular injury is suspected. Patients with soft signs of vascular injury and an ABI <0.9 usually need arteriography to rule out or verify vascular damage. This is performed as soon as possible. Before the patient is sent to the angiosuite other injuries need to be taken into account and the priority of management discussed. Ischemic legs should be given higher priority than, for example, skeletal and soft tissue injury, and temporary restoration of blood flow can be achieved by shunting.

Patients with an ABI >0.9 and a normal physical examination (little suspicion of vascular injury) can be monitored in the ward. Repeated examinations of the patient's clinical status are important and hourly assessment of pulses and ABI the first 4–6 h are warranted. If the ABI deteriorates to a value <0.9 or if pulses disappear, angiography should be carried out.

9.5.1.3 Angiography Findings

Operative treatment and restoration of blood flow are done as soon as possible if the angiography shows arterial occlusion in the femoral, popliteal, or at least two calf arteries in proximity to the traumatized area. It should be kept in mind that occlusion of the popliteal artery is detrimental for distal perfusion and is associated with a high risk for amputation due to a long ischemia time. Patients with popliteal occlusion should therefore be taken immediately to the operating room. Debate is ongoing whether one patent calf artery in an injured leg is sufficient to allow nonoperative treatment. Some reports have found that as long as one of the tibial vessels is intact, there is no difference in limb loss or foot problems during follow-up between operative and nonoperative treatment. Our recommendation, however, is to try to restore perfusion if more than one of the calf arteries is obstructed.

If combined with ischemic symptoms or signs of embolization, angiography findings of intimal flaps, minor narrowing of an artery, or minor pseudoanuerysm (<5 mm in diameter) should also be treated. Endovascular stenting is then a good alternative to operative treatment. Expectancy could be favorable for asymptomatic patients with normal ABI. Such occult arterial injuries appear to have an uneventful course and late occlusion is extremely rare. The occasional pseudoaneurysm that will enlarge with time appears to benefit from later repair.

9.5.1.4 Primary Amputation

In most circumstances, but not always, it is reasonable to repair injured vessels. For a few patients, however, primary amputation is a better option. This is often a difficult decision. Primary amputation is favorable for the patient if the leg is massacred or if the duration of ischemia is very long (>12 h) and appears to be irreversible in the clinical examination (Chapter 10, p. 123). Primary amputation may also be considered for certain patients: multitrauma patients, patients with severe comorbid disease, and those in whom the leg was already paralyzed at the time of injury. Extensive nerve damage, lack of soft tissue to cover the wound, and duration of ischemia >6 h support primary amputation for these patient groups.

There are scoring systems, such as the Mangled Extremity Severity Score (MESS), to aid in making the decision to amputate a leg or an arm. For example, a patient over 50 years old with persistent hypotension and a cool paralyzed distal leg after high-energy trauma should have the leg amputated according to MESS. It must be stressed, however, that repair of both venous and arterial injuries is superior for most patients. The MESS score is described in Chapter 3 (p. 36).

9.5.2 Operation

Surgical treatment of vascular injuries in the leg usually proceeds in a particular order common for most patients. First the patient is scrubbed, anesthetized, and prepared for surgery. The next step is to achieve proximal control. Occasionally, control of the bleeding by manual compression with a gloved hand needs to be maintained throughout these first two steps. Proximal control is followed by measures to achieve distal control, often accomplished during exploration of the wound. Finally, the vessels are repaired and the wound covered with soft tissue. When the patient has other injuries that motivate urgent treatment, or has fractures in the leg that need to be surgically repaired, this last step can be delayed while perfusion to the distal leg is maintained by a shunt temporarily bypassing the injured area.

9.5.2.1 Preoperative Preparation

The patient is placed on a surgical table that allows x-ray penetration. If not administered previously, infection prophylaxis treatment is started. The entire injured extremity is scrubbed with the foot draped in a transparent plastic bag. A very good marginal of the sterile field is essential because incisions need to be placed much more proximal than the wound to achieve proximal control. The contralateral leg should also be scrubbed and draped to allow harvest of veins for grafts. The venous system in the injured leg should be kept intact if possible. If a patient is in shock and the bleeding is difficult to control, it is recommended to delay inducing the anesthesia until just before the operation begins in order to avoid increased bleeding and an accentuated drop in systemic blood pressure due to loss of adrenergic activity.

NOTE

It is usually wise to achieve proximal control through a separate incision before exploring the wounded area.

9.5.2.2 Proximal Control

In patients with injuries proximal to the femoral vessels, control is achieved through an incision in the abdominal fossa. The common or external iliac artery can then be exposed retroperitoneally and secured. Proximal control for injuries in the thigh, proximal to the poplital fossa, is usually obtained by exposing the common femoral artery and its branches in the groin. Popliteal vessel trauma can be controlled by exposing the distal superficial femoral artery or the proximal popliteal artery through a medial incision above the knee. This is not too difficult, and the principles follow the outline given in the Technical Tips box. Inflow control for calf vessel injuries is reached by exposing the popliteal artery below the knee.

If there is no ongoing bleeding when the artery is exposed a vessel-loop is applied. Clamping should be postponed until later. If bleeding is brisk and continuous, however, the clamp is placed right away. Clamping should be attempted even if the bleeding appears to be mainly venous in origin. Arterial clamping often diminishes such bleedings substantially.

An alternative way to achieve proximal control of distal femoral, popliteal, and calf vessels is to use a cuff. A padded cuff, the width in accordance with the leg circumference, is then wrapped around the leg well above the wounded area before scrubbing and draping. In the thigh a 20-cm wide cuff is often suitable. It is important to have at least 10 cm from the lower edge of the cuff to the wound to allow prolongation of incisions if necessary. The cuff is inflated if bleeding starts during exploration. For distal injuries this often works well and may spare the patient one surgical wound.

NOTE
Tourniquet occlusion is a good option for proximal control of distal injuries.

TECHNICAL TIPS
Exposure of Different Vessel Segments in the Leg

■ **Common or External Iliac Arteries,** Fig. 9.1
a A skin incision 5 cm above and parallel to the inguinal ligament is used. This incision allows exposure of all vascular segments from the external iliac up to the aortic bifurcation.
b The muscles are split in the direction of the fibers. Dissection is totally retroperitoneal, with attention to the ureter crossing the vessels in this region. Be careful with the iliac vein, which is separated from the artery by only a thin tissue layer. Exposure of the proximal common iliac artery and the aortic bifurcation is facilitated by a table-fixed self-retaining retractor (i.e., Martin arm).

■ **Femoral Artery in the Groin,** Fig. 9.2
a A longitudinal skin incision starting 1–2 cm cranial to the inguinal skin fold and continued lateral to the artery is used to avoid the inguinal lymph nodes. A common mistake is to place the incision too far caudally, which usually means the dissection is taking place distal to the deep femoral.
b The dissection is continued sharply with the knife straight down to the fascia lateral to the lymph nodes and is then angulated 90° medially to reach the area over the artery. It should then be palpable. Lymph nodes should be avoided to minimize the risk for infection and development of seroma. The fascia is incised, and the anterior and lateral surfaces of the artery are approached.

c At this stage the anatomy is often unclear regarding the relation of branches to the common femoral artery. Encircle the exposed artery with a vessel-loop as described in Chapter 15, and gently lift the artery. Continue dissection until the bifurcation into superficial and deep femoral artery is identified. Its location varies from high up under the inguinal ligament up to 10 cm further down. At this stage, the surgeon must decide whether exposure and clamping of the common femoral are enough. This is usually the case for proximal control in trauma distally in the leg. In acute ischemia it is more common that the entire bifurcation needs to be exposed.

During the continued dissection, attention must be given to important branches that should be controlled and protected from iatrogenic injuries. These are, in particular, the circumflex iliac artery on the dorsal aspect of the common femoral artery and the deep femoral vein crossing over the anterior aspect of the deep femoral artery just after its bifurcation. To provide a safe and good exposure of the deep femoral to a level below its first bifurcation, this vein must be divided and suture-ligated. Partial division of the inguinal ligament is occasionally needed for satisfactory exposure.

▼

TECHNICAL TIPS
Exposure of Different Vessel Segments in the Leg (continued)

■ **Superficial Femoral Artery,** Fig. 9.3

A skin incision is made along the dorsal aspect of the sartorius muscle at a midthigh level. It is important to avoid injuries to the greater saphenous vein, which usually is located in the posterior flap of the incision. The incision can be elongated as needed. After the deep fascia is opened and the sartorius muscle is retracted anteriorly, the femoral artery is found and can be mobilized. Division of the adductor tendon is sometimes required for exposure.

■ **Popliteal Artery Above the Knee,** Fig. 9.4

a The knee is supported on a sterile, draped pillow. The skin incision is started at the medial aspect of the femoral condyle and follows the anterior border of the sartorius muscle 10–15 cm in a proximal direction. Protect the greater saphenous vein and the saphenous nerve during dissection down to the fascia. After dividing the fascia longitudinally, continue the dissection in the groove between the sartorius and gracilis muscles, which leads to the fat in the popliteal fossa.

a The popliteal artery and adjacent veins and nerve are then, without further division of muscles, easily found and separated in the anterior aspect of the fossa.

■ **Popliteal Artery Below the Knee,** Fig. 9.5

a A sterile pillow or pad is placed under the distal femur. The incision is placed 1 or 2 cm posterior to the medial border of the tibia, starting at the tibial tuberosity and extending 10–12 cm distally. Subcutaneous fat and fascia are sharply divided, with caution to the greater saphenous vein.

b The popliteal fossa is reached by retracting the gastrocnemius muscle dorsally. The deep fascia is divided and the artery usually easier to identifiy. Occasionally, pes anserinus must be divided for adequate exposure. The popliteal artery is often located just anterior to the nerve and in close contact with the popliteal vein and crossing branches from concomitant veins. If it is necessary to expose the more distal parts of the popliteal artery, the soleus muscle has to be divided and partly separated from the posterior border of the tibia.

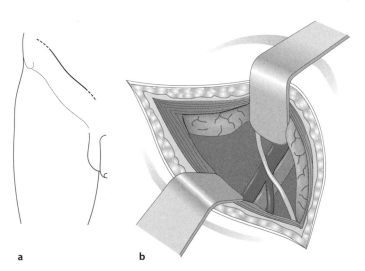

Fig. 9.1. Exposure of common or external iliac arteries. Note the ureter crossing the arteries anteriorly

a   b

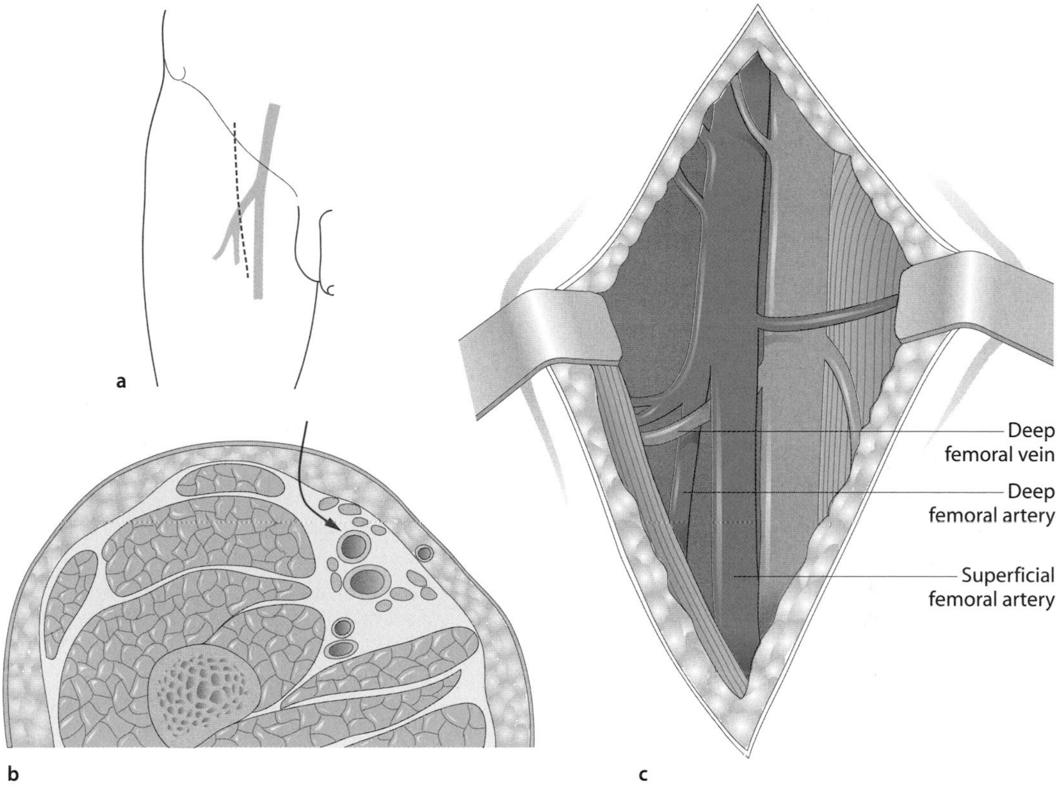

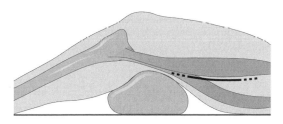

Fig. 9.2. Exposure of femoral artery in the groin

Deep
femoral vein

Deep
femoral artery

Superficial
femoral artery

Fig. 9.3. Incision for exposure of the superficial femoral artery

■ 9.5.2.3 Distal Control and Exploration

Distal control is achieved by distal elongation of the incision used to explore the site of injury. Through this incision careful dissection in intact tissue distal to the injured area usually reveals the injured artery. When it is identified and found to be not completely transected, a vessel-loop is positioned around it. If the artery is cut, a vascular clamp is applied on the stump. It is also possible to gain distal control during the exploration of the injured area, but dissection may be tricky because of hematoma, edema, and distorted anatomy. Usually the backbleeding from the distal artery is minimal and does not disturb visualization during dissection. Simultaneous venous bleeding that emerges from major veins must also be controlled. This can be done by balloon occlusion or clamps. The latter should be used with caution and closed as little as possible.

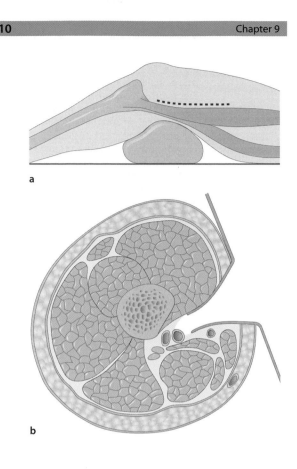

a

b

Fig. 9.4. Exposure of popliteal artery above the knee

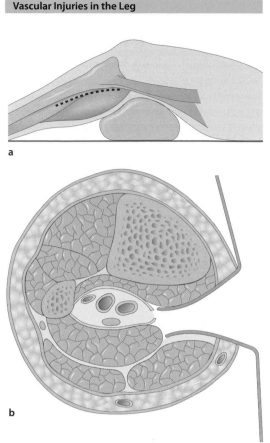

a

b

Fig. 9.5. Exposure of popliteal artery below the knee

When control is obtained the wound is explored and the site of vessel injury identified. The best way is to follow the artery proximally from where the artery was exposed for distal control. Of course, any foreign materials encountered need to be removed. The injured artery should be explored in both directions until a normal arterial wall is reached. Several centimeters of free vessels are needed. Side branches are controlled using a double loop of suture with a hanging mosquito or by small vascular clamps (see Chapter 15, p. 181). Thrombosed arteries usually have a hematoma in the vessel wall giving it a dark blue color. Such parts need to be cut out and the vessel edges trimmed before shunting or repair. For penetrating injuries all parts of the vascular wall that are lacerated must be excised to ensure that the intima will be enclosed in the suture line during repair. After this procedure the vessel can be shunted or repaired.

Finally, other parts of the wound are explored and all devitalized skin and muscle tissue is excised. Injured small adjacent veins should be ligated and all larger veins, such as the femoral veins and the popliteal vein, must be repaired.

9.5.2.4 Shunting

Insertion of a temporary shunt to restore distal perfusion is sensible if the vascular injury appears to require more extensive repair than a simple suture or an end-to-end anastomsis. Shunting provides the time needed to either perform a vascular reconstruction, including harvesting of a vein graft from the uninjured leg, or to wait for help. Shunting can also be valuable when patients have other injuries that need attention or when leg fractures must be repositioned to give the appropriate vascular graft length. In patients with fractures shunting allows both repositioning and fixation without increasing the risk of ischemic damage.

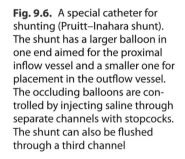

Fig. 9.6. A special catheter for shunting (Pruitt–Inahara shunt). The shunt has a larger balloon in one end aimed for the proximal inflow vessel and a smaller one for placement in the outflow vessel. The occluding balloons are controlled by injecting saline through separate channels with stopcocks. The shunt can also be flushed through a third channel

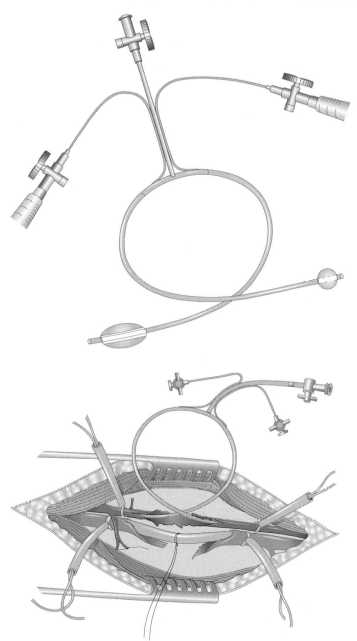

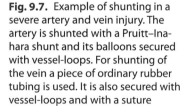

Fig. 9.7. Example of shunting in a severe artery and vein injury. The artery is shunted with a Pruitt–Inahara shunt and its balloons secured with vessel-loops. For shunting of the vein a piece of ordinary rubber tubing is used. It is also secured with vessel-loops and with a suture

A novel vascular reconstruction seldom tolerates the forces required for reposition of fractures. When perfusion is restored by a shunt the surgeon has plenty of time to carefully explore the wound and other injuries. When a shunt is used for distal perfusion while other procedures are performed, it is important to check its function at least every 30 min.

The principles of vascular shunting are simple. Specially designed shunts can be used if available; examples are Pruitt–Inahara and Javid. Most have inflatable balloons in both ends for occlusion and side channels with stopcocks through which the function of the shunt can be tested (Figs. 9.6, 9.7). The side holes also enable infusion of a heparinized solution and contrast for fluoroscopy. The extra channels can be used to draw blood during the operation. It is not, however, necessary to use manufactured shunts. Any kind of sterile plastic or rubber tubing is sufficient. It is then important to use dimensions of the tube in accordance with the artery's inner diameter. The tube is cut into suitable lengths and the edges carefully trimmed with scalpel and scissors to avoid damage when inserted. The tube is positioned and secured with vessel loops that abolish the space between the artery and tube to manage bleeding. A loosely applied suture around the middle part of the shunt can be used to secure it. It is advantageous to simultaneously shunt concomitant vein injuries – at least the femoral and popliteal veins – to avoid swelling and to facilitate distal flow.

9.5.2.5 Vessel Repair

While we advocate repairing both the artery and the vein, we do not favor reconstructing the injured vein before the artery. If both can be mended within a reasonable timeframe we recommend that the most difficult reconstruction is performed first. If, however, the artery is shunted it may be advantageous to start with the vein to achieve optimal outflow as soon as possible. Some vascular surgeons favor vein ligature as a general principle because of the potential risk for embolization from vein segments that thrombose after repair.

NOTE
Popliteal occlusions should be managed quickly because of the high risk of amputation in case of delayed treatment.

Arterial Injuries

In general, all injured arteries should be repaired. Sometimes, when necessary in order to save the patient's life or when interruption of an artery does not influence blood flow to the leg, the injured vessel may be ligated. The former is extremely uncommon, but the decision is difficult when it arises. As an aid we have listed in Table 9.3 the amputation rates, as obtained from the literature, following ligation of vessels. Among proximal vessels, only branches from the deep femoral artery, but not the main branch, can be ligated without morbidity. Distally, we recommend repair of at least two calf arteries to be on the safe side, but it is

Table 9.3. Amputation frequencies after ligature of different arteries

Vessel ligated	Amputation rate
Common iliac artery	54%
External iliac artery	47%
Common femoral artery	81%
Superficial femoral artery	55%
Popliteal artery	73%

possible to leave two interrupted, provided the remaining vessel is not the peroneal artery.

Before definitive repair the surgeon must be sure that the inflow and outflow vascular beds remain open and are free of clots. Liberal use of Fogarty catheters is therefore wise. The technique is described in Chapter 10 (p. 126). If the backbleeding is questionable, intraoperative angiography should be performed to make sure the outflow tract is free of clots. Local heparinization, described in Chapter 15 (p. 181), is always indicated. Systemic heparinization can be used for selected patients without other injuries considered to have a low risk for continued bleeding from the wound after debridement. If the foot's appearance or intraoperative angiography suggests microembolization, local thrombolysis can be tried as described in Chapter 10 (p. 127).

The goal for repair is to permanently restore continuity of the artery without stenosis or tension. The type of injury determines the choice of technique. It varies from a couple of vascular sutures to reconstruction with a patch, interposition, or a bypass grafting. Lateral suture for repair of minor lesions, including patching, is described in Chapter 15 (p. 183). Bypass techniques are beyond the scope of this book, and detailed descriptions can be found in other vascular surgery textbooks.

A graft is usually needed, and only occasionally can an end-to-end anastomosis be performed without tension. It is always better to use an interposition graft or a bypass to avoid what is even perceived as insignificant tension because anastomotic rupture and graft necrosis may occur when leg swelling and movements pull the arterial ends further apart postoperatively. The major bleeding that can result from this may even be fatal.

An autologous vein is always the preferred graft material. Vein is more infection resistant than synthetic materials and is more flexible. It allows both elongation and vasodilatation to adjust variations in flow requirements. The great saphenous vein from the contralateral leg is the primary choice for a graft. It is a serious mistake to use the great saphenous vein from the traumatized leg if the deep vein is also injured or if injury is suspected. Interruption of the saphenous vein with obstructed concomitant deep veins will rapidly cause severe distal swelling of the leg and graft occlusion within days. The vein can be harvested at a level in the leg where the saphenous vein diameter fits the artery that needs to be repaired. A graft slightly larger than the artery should be obtained if possible. For common femoral artery lesions, two pieces of saphenous vein, both open longitudinally and then sutured together, might be required. An option is to use arm veins as graft material. If veins not are available expanded polytetrafluoroethylene (ePTFE) is the second choice. The main reasons not to use it are the slightly higher risks for postoperative graft occlusion and infection.

Venous injuries

Most venous injuries are exposed when the wound is explored. While vein ligature may lead to leg swelling, it rarely causes ischemia or amputation. On the other hand, the only benefit of vein ligature is rapid bleeding control and a reduced operating time. Major veins can therefore be ligated to save the life of an unstable patient. If possible, however, most veins should be repaired, especially the popliteal and the common femoral veins. Calf veins can be ligated without morbidity. In patients with combined injuries, both the vein and the artery should be repaired to enhance the function of the arterial reconstruction. Control of bleedings can be achieved by fingers or a "strawberry" or "peanut" to compress the vein proximal and distal to the injured site, or by using gentle vascular clamps. A continuous running suture, almost without traction in the suture line, is often sufficient to close a stab wound. When the vein is more extensively damaged, a patch or an interposition graft may be needed for repair. As with arteries, it is important to match the caliber of the interposition graft and the injured vein. Veins without blood are collapsed, so it is easy to underestimate

their size. An autologous vein is preferred over synthetic materials.

9.5.2.6 Finishing the Operation

After the vascular reconstruction is finished the resulting improvement in distal perfusion should be checked. This is indicated as well-perfused skin in the foot and palpable pulses. If there is any doubt about the result control angiography should be performed. Preferably, it is done from the proximal control site to enable visualization of all anastomoses. If problems are revealed the reconstruction must be redone and distal clots extracted as previously described. While vascular spasm is rare and should not be regarded as the main explanation for lack of distal blood flow, injection of 1–2 ml papaverine into the graft can also be tried.

After vascular repair all devitalized tissue and foreign material should be removed to reduce the risk of postoperative infection. Grafts and vessels should be covered with healthy tissue by loosely adapting it with interrupted absorbable sutures. For injuries with massive tissue loss it may be impossible to cover the graft. This increases the risk for postoperative anastomotic necrosis and rupture. Split or partial skin grafts or biological dressings can be used to prevent this. Occasionally it may be better to perform a bypass through healthy tissue, thus avoiding the traumatized area, to minimize graft infection and postoperative complications.

9.5.3 Endovascular Treatment

Endovascular treatment of vascular injuries to leg vessels is attractive because it provides a way to achieve proximal control, reduce ischemia time, and simplify complex procedures. There is not a lot of experience – at least not reported in the literature – with endovascular treatment. Some centers have reported successful semielective treatment of pseudoaneurysms and arteriovenous fistulas in the groin. Small patient series have been published on embolization of bleeding branches to the deep femoral artery and stent graft control of small lacerations in the femoral arteries. We have only treated occasional patients this way so far.

Endovascular treatment will probably be an option for many patients with soft signs of vascular injury, who will undergo angiography and then will be found to have a minor bleeding, a pseudoaneurysm, a fistula, or an intimal flap. The possibilities of considering endovascular repair for patients with hard signs of vascular injury to the legs will depend on logistics and the organization of a hospital's endovascular team. With around-the-clock availability, patients with less severe distal ischemia may be subjected to angiography with possibilities for endovascular treatment in mind. Patients with penetrating injuries that are actively bleeding may undergo balloon occlusion of a proximal artery to accomplish control and then be transferred to the operating room for repair. In other hospitals where an endovascular team is not available during weekends, angiography is skipped in some patients with soft signs, and they are treated with an open procedure and intraoperative angiography instead. But it is likely that endovascular treatment will be the treatment of choice for a significant proportion of patients in the near future.

9.5.4 Management After Treatment

As for most vascular procedures, the risk for bleeding and graft thrombosis of the reconstructed artery is higher during the first 24 h after the operation. Postoperative monitoring of limb perfusion, including inspection of foot skin and wounds and palpation of pulses, is necessary at least every 30 min for the first 6 h. If pulses are difficult to ascertain, ankle pressure should be measured. Loss of pulses or an abrupt drop in pressure indicate that reoperation may be required, even when the graft appears to be patent either clinically or on duplex scanning. As for acute leg ischemia caused by thrombosis, there is also a substantial risk for compartment syndrome. Particularly when the ischemia duration has been long, this risk is considerable, and it is important to examine calf muscles for signs of compartment syndrome. This assessment includes motor function, tenderness, and palpation of the muscle compartments in the calf. Findings that may suggest fasciotomy are listed in Table 9.4

For most patients administration of dextran or low molecular weight heparin is indicated to avoid postoperative thrombosis. This is especially im-

Table 9.4. Medical history and clinical findings suggesting that fasciotomy may be needed

Severe ischemia lasting longer than 4–6 h
Preoperative shock
Firm/hard muscle compartment when palpated
Decreased sensibility and/or motor function
Compartmental pressure >30 mmHg
Pain out of proportion localized distal to the vascular injury

portant for patients with both venous and arterial reconstruction. Patients who have been subjected to venous ligation need extra attention and measures against limb swelling. Antibiotic treatment started preoperatively or intraoperatively is usually continued after the operation. We use a combination of benzylpenicillin and isoxazolyl penicillin to cover streptococci, clostridia, and staphylococci.

9.6 Results and Outcome

Mortality after isolated vascular injuries in the legs is very low, ranging from 0% to 3% in most series. The few deaths reported were due to infection and sepsis, underscoring the importance of careful tissue debridement and graft coverage. For solitary vascular injuries, amputation rates are also low. It has to be remembered that important nerves are located adjacent to the vessels and often are simultaneously severely damaged. This contributes to long-term disability. In most studies, arterial patency is very high, while venous reconstructions tend to thrombose at a much higher frequency. Although some authors have argued that venous repair is therefore unnecessary, we believe it improves patency of the arterial graft. Fractures, especially open ones, in combination with arterial injury have less encouraging long-term results. In most reports the incidence of primary as well as secondary amputation is higher when fractures are combined with vascular and nerve injuries. In one study the primary and secondary amputation rates were 20% and 52%, respectively, during a follow-up of 5.6 years. There was a 30% long-term disability rate for salvaged limbs in the same study, all related to poor recovery of neurological function. Although it is clear that popliteal injuries, combined injuries with femoral fractures, delayed repair >6 h, and injuries treated in patients in shock have a much higher amputation rate, the results may be less pessimistic than the results in the literature. For multitrauma patients outcomes of vascular injury in the leg are hard to come by.

■ 9.7 Fasciotomy

When the compartment pressure is clearly increased or when there is a risk of developing increased pressure, fasciotomy of muscular compartments distal to a vascular injury should be performed in association with the vascular repair. Factors suggesting an increased pressure are listed in Table 9.4. The technique for decompression of the four compartments in the lower leg is described in the Technical Tips box.

TECHNICAL TIPS
Fasciotomy of the Calf Compartments (Two Incisions)

■ Medial Incision
A 15–20-cm-long skin incision, starting slightly below the midpoint of the calf and downwards parallel to and 2–3 cm dorsally of the medial border of the tibia, is used to decompress the deep and superficial posterior muscle compartments (Fig. 9.8). It is important to avoid injury to the great saphenous vein. Sharp division of skin and subcutaneous fat reaches the fascia. The skin and subcutaneous fat is mobilized en bloc anteriorly and posteriorly to expose it enough to provide access to the compartments. The fascia is then opened in a proximal direction and distally down toward the malleolus under the soleus muscle. At this level, the soleus muscle has no attachments to the tibia, and the deep posterior compartment is more superficial and easier to access. Through the same skin incision, the fascia of the superficial posterior muscle compartment is cleaved 2–3 cm dorsally and parallel to the former. A long straight pair of scissors with blunt points is used to cut the fascia using a distinct continuous movement in the distal direction, down to a level of 5 cm above the malleoli and proximally along the entire fascia. ▼

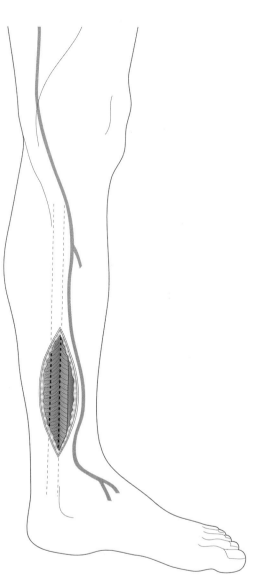

Fig. 9.8. Incision and exposure for fasciotomy of posterior compartments. The *posterior dotted line* indicates fasciotomy incision for the superficial compartment and the *anterior dotted line* for the deep compartment

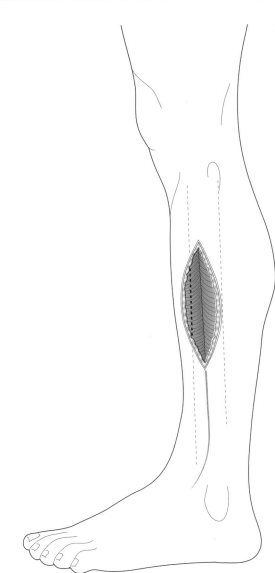

Fig. 9.9. Incision for fasciotomy of anterior and lateral compartments. Through the demonstrated skin incision, long incisions are made along the *dotted lines* in the fascia. Caution must be taken with the peroneal nerve

■ Lateral Incision

The skin incision for fasciotomy of the lateral and anterior muscle compartments is oriented anterior to and in parallel with the fibula. The dorsal position of the lateral compartment, however, often requires more extensive mobilization of the subcutaneous fat to reach it. The superficial peroneal nerve is located anteriorly under the fascia and exits the compartment through the anterior aspect of the fascia distally in the calf. To preserve this nerve, direct the scissors dorsally when making the fasciotomy in both directions. (See Fig. 9.9.)

Unless the swelling is very extensive, 2-0 prolene intradermal suture is loosely placed to enable wound closure later (Fig. 9.10). It is important to leave long suture ends at both sides to allow wound edge separation the first postoperative days. The skin incisions are left open with moist dressings.

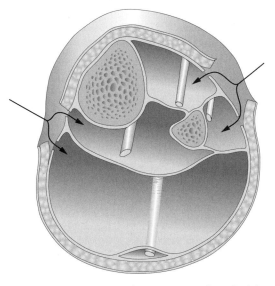

Fig. 9.10. Cross-section demonstrating the principles for decompression of all four muscle compartments in the calf through a medial and a lateral incision. The location of major nerve bundles in the different compartments is indicated

9.8 Iatrogenic Vascular Injuries to the Legs

Iatrogenic vascular injuries occur either in connection with other surgical procedures or as a complication to groin catheterization for angiography, percutaneous coronary intervention, and other endovascular procedures. The latter constitutes the main part. In this book, bleeding and pseudoaneurysms that occur after angiography are covered in Chapter 14.

Vascular injury during surgery is also quite common. The risk for vessel trauma during operations varies with the type of procedure. Certain procedures are also more prone to cause vascular injury (Table 9.5), and vascular procedures are the ones most frequently associated with vascular injury. Suspicious signs of vascular injury during surgery are sudden bleeding that fills the operative field and problems maintaining the systemic blood pressure. This is exemplified by major bleeding occurring behind retractors or in a field previously dissected during abdominal aortic aneurysm surgery. When the bleeding area is identified, it is controlled by manual compression. It is wise to always call for help when major bleeding is suspected. More hands facilitate repair, and realizing that one has caused a severe vascular injury may generate stress and distract the surgeon from accomplishing vascular repair.

The technique used for vascular repair is the same as for all other vascular injuries. While maintaining compression, proximal and distal control is created by careful dissection of the vessels around the suspected injury site. The vessel is then clamped or controlled by finger or swab compression. The traumatized vessel is then repaired. For iatrogenic injuries this often means just a few sutures; only rarely is more complex repair needed.

There are also specially designed instruments for controlling vessels – especially veins – enough to allow suturing without needing extensive exposure to achieve control. One consists of a ring 2–3 cm in diameter welded at a 75° angle to a handle. The ring is placed around the injured vein and held in place, thereby controlling the bleeding. This device is particularly helpful for iliac vein bleedings that occur during gynecologic, urologic, and rectal cancer operations. Multiple vessel injuries are not uncommon and perseverance is often needed to repair all vessels before the original operation can proceed.

Further Reading

Dennis JW, Frykberg ER, Veldenz HC, et al.Validation of nonoperative management of occult vascular injuries and accuracy of physical examination alone in penetrating extremity trauma: 5- to 10-year follow up. J Trauma 1998; 44(2):243–252

Hafez HM, Woolgar J, Robbs JV. Lower extremity arterial injury: results of 550 cases and review of risk factors associated with limb loss. J Vasc Surg 2001; 33(6):1212–1219

Hood DB, Weaver FA, Yellin AE. Changing perspectives in the diagnosis of peripheral vascular trauma. Semin Vasc Surg 1998; 11(4):255–260

Modrall JG, Weaver FA, Yellin AE. Vascular considerations in extremity trauma. Orthop Clin North Am 1993; 24(3):557–563

Nair R, Abdool-Carrim AT, Robbs JV. Gunshot injuries of the popliteal artery. Br J Surg 2000; 87(5):602

Rich NM. Management of venous trauma. Surg Clin North Am 1988; 68(4):809–821

Rowe VL, Salim A, Lipham J, et al. Shank vessel injuries. Surg Clin North Am 2002; 82(1):91–104

Snyder WH 3rd. Popliteal and shank arterial injury. Surg Clin North Am 1988; 68(4):787–807

Table 9.5. Examples of procedures associated with iatrogenic vascular injury (*PCI* percutaneous coronary intervention)

Procedure	Vessel injured
PCI/angiography	Common femoral, external iliac, deep femoral arteries
Knee arthroplasty	Popliteal artery and vein
Hip arthroplasty	Common femoral
Stripping of saphenous vein	Common femoral vein (groin arteries)

Acute Leg Ischemia

10

CONTENTS

■ 10.1 Summary

- It is important to evaluate the severity of ischemia.
- If the leg is immediately threatened, operation cannot be delayed.
- If the leg is viable, there is no benefit of an emergency operation.
- Before the operation it is vital to consider the etiology of the occlusion, to be prepared to perform a distal vascular reconstruction, and to treat heart and pulmonary failure if present.

■ 10.2 Background

■ 10.2.1 Background

Acute leg ischemia is associated with a great risk for amputation and death. The age of the patients is high, and to some extent acute leg ischemia can be considered an end-of-life disease. Patients' symptoms and the clinical signs of the afflicted leg vary. Sometimes grave ischemia immediately threatens limb viability, such as after a large embolization to a healthy vascular bed. Other times the symptoms are less dramatic, appearing as onset of rest pain in a patient with claudication. This is usually due to thrombosis of a previously stenosed artery.

Table 10.1. Incidence of acute leg ischemia

Country	Year	Surveyed population size	Population	Yearly incidence per 100,000 inhabitants
Sweden	1965–1983	1.5 million	All treated or amputated, >70 years old	125 (men) 150 (women)
USA	2000		All hospitalized	95
Sweden	1990–1994	2.0 million	All treated	60 (men) 77 (Women)
United Kingdom	1995	0.5 million	All diagnosed	14–16

It is the severity of ischemia that determines management and treatment. To minimize the risk for amputation or persistent dysfunction it is important to rapidly restore perfusion if an extremity is immediately threatened. When the leg shows signs of severe ischemia but is clearly viable, it is equally important to thoroughly evaluate and optimize the patient before any intervention is initiated. These basic management principles are generally applicable. Accordingly, we recommend "management by severity" rather than "management by etiology" (thrombosis versus embolus) but recognize that the latter can also be an effective strategy.

10.2.2 Magnitude of the Problem

It is difficult to find accurate incidence figures on acute leg ischemia. Data from some reports are given in Table 10.1. The numbers listed do not include conservatively treated patients or those whose legs were amputated as a primary procedure. The incidence increases with age and is seen with equal frequency in men and women. Regardless, the frequency indicates that it is a very common problem.

10.2.3 Pathogenesis and Etiology

10.2.3.1 Pathogenesis

Acute leg ischemia is caused by a sudden deterioration of perfusion to the distal parts of the leg. While the abrupt inhibition of blood flow causes the ischemia, its consequences are variable because acute leg ischemia is multifactorial in origin. Hypercoagulable states, cardiac failure, and dehy-

dration predispose the blood for thrombosis and make the tissue more vulnerable to decreased perfusion. Besides the fact that a healthy leg is more vulnerable than one accustomed to low perfusion, it is unknown what determines the viability of the tissue. The most important factor is probably the duration of ischemia. The type of tissue affected also influences viability. In the leg, the skin is more ischemia-tolerant than skeletal muscle.

10.2.3.2 Embolus and Thrombosis

The etiology of the occlusion is not what determines the management process. It is, however, of importance when choosing therapy. Embolus is usually best treated by embolectomy, whereas arterial thrombosis is preferably resolved by thrombolysis, percutaneous transluminal angioplasty (PTA), or a vascular reconstruction. The reason for this difference is that emboli often obstruct a relatively healthy vascular bed, whereas thrombosis occurs in an already diseased atherosclerotic artery. Consequently, emboli more often cause immediate threatening ischemia and require urgent restoration of blood flow. Thrombosis, on the other hand, occurs in a leg with previous arterial insufficiency with well-developed collaterals. In the latter case it is important not only to solve the acute thrombosis but also to get rid of the cause. It must be kept in mind that emboli can be lodged in atherosclerotic arteries as well, which then makes embolectomy more difficult.

Table 10.2 summarizes typical findings in the medical history and physical examination that suggest thrombosis or embolism. Many risk factors, such as cardiac disease, are common for both embolization and thrombosis. Atrial fibrillation and a recent (less than 4 weeks) myocardial infarction with intramural thrombus are the two domi-

Table 10.2. History and clinical findings differentiating the etiology of acute ischemia

Thrombosis	Embolism
Previous claudication	No previous symptoms of arterial insufficiency
No source of emboli	Obvious source of emboli (arterial fibrillation, myocardial infarction)
Long history (days to weeks)	Sudden onset (hours to days)
Less severe ischemia	Severe ischemia
Lack of pulses in the contralateral leg	Normal pulses in the contralateral leg
Positive signs of chronic ischemia	No signs of chronic ischemia

nating sources for emboli (80–90%). Other possible origins are aneurysms and atherosclerotic plaques located proximal to the occluded vessel. The latter are often associated with microembolization (discussed later) but may also cause larger emboli.

Plaque rupture, immobilization, and hypercoagulability are the main causes of acute thrombosis. Severe cardiac failure, dehydration, and bleeding are less common causes. Hypoperfusion due to such conditions can easily turn an extremity with longstanding slightly compromised perfusion into acute ischemia.

10.3 Clinical Presentation

10.3.1 Medical History

The typical patient with acute leg ischemia is old and has had a recent myocardial infarction. He or she describes a sudden onset of symptoms – a few hours of pain, coldness, loss of sensation, and poor mobility in the foot and calf. Accordingly, all signs of threatened leg viability are displayed. The event is most likely an embolization, and the patient needs urgent surgery. Unfortunately, such patients are unusual among those who are admitted for acute leg ischemia. The history is often variable, and sometimes it is difficult to decide even the time of onset of symptoms.

It is important to obtain a detailed medical history to reveal any underlying conditions or lesions that may have caused the ischemia. Moreover, identifying and treating comorbidities may improve the outcome after surgery or thrombolysis.

10.3.2 Clinical Signs and Symptoms

The symptoms and signs of acute ischemia are often summarized as the "five Ps": pain, pallor, pulselessness, paresthesia, and paralysis. Besides being helpful for establishing diagnosis, careful evaluation of the five Ps is useful for assessing the severity of ischemia. Sometimes a sixth P's is used – poikolothermia, meaning a low skin temperature that does not vary with the environment.

Pain: For the typical patient, as the one described above, the pain is severe, continuous, and localized in the foot and toes. Its intensity is unrelated to the severity of ischemia. For instance, it is less pronounced when the ischemia is so severe that the nerve fibers transmitting the sensation of pain are damaged. Patients with diabetes often have neuropathy and a decreased sensation of pain.

Pallor: The ischemic leg is pale or white initially, but when ischemia aggravates the color turns to cyanotic blue. This cyanosis is caused by vessel dilatation and desaturation of hemoglobin in the skin and is induced by acidic metabolites in combination with stagnant blood flow. Consequently, cyanosis is a graver sign of ischemia than pallor.

Pulselessness: A palpable pulse in a peripheral artery means that the flow in the vessel is sufficient to give a pulse that is synchronous with vessel dilatation, which can be palpated with the fingers. In general, palpable pulses in the foot therefore exclude severe leg ischemia. When there is a fresh thrombus, pulses can be felt in spite of an occlusion, so this general principle must be applied with caution. Palpation of pulses can be used to identify the level of obstruction and is facilitated by comparing the presence of pulses at the same level in the contralateral leg.

When the examiner is not convinced that palpable pulses are present, distal blood pressures must be measured. It is prudent to always measure the ankle blood pressure. This is a simple way to verify ischemia and the measurement can be used to grade the severity and serve as a baseline for comparison with repeated examinations during the course of treatment. (This will be discussed further later.) The continuous-wave (CW) Doppler instrument does not give information about the magnitude of flow because it registers only flow velocities in the vessel. Therefore, an audible signal with a CW Doppler is not equivalent to a palpable pulse, and a severely ischemic leg can have audible Doppler signals.

NOTE

In acute leg ischemia, the principle use of CW Doppler is to measure ankle blood pressure.

Paresthesia: The thin nerve fibers conducting impulses from light touch are very sensitive to ischemia and are damaged soon after perfusion is interrupted. Pain fibers are less ischemia-sensitive. Accordingly, the most precise test of sensibility is to lightly touch the skin with the fingertips, alternating between the affected and the healthy leg. It is a common mistake to believe that the skin has been touched too gently when the patient actually has impaired sensitivity. The examiner then may proceed to pinching and poking the skin with a needle. Such tests of pain fibers evaluate a much later stage of ischemic damage. The anatomic localization of impaired sensation is sometimes related to which nerves are involved. Frequently, however, it does not follow nerve distribution areas and is circumferential and most severe distally. Numbness and tingling are other symptoms of ischemic disturbance of nerve function.

Paralysis: Loss of motor function in the leg is initially caused by ischemic destruction of motor nerve fibers and at later stages the ischemia directly affects muscle tissue. When palpated, ischemic muscles are tender and have a spongy feeling. Accordingly, the entire leg can become paretic after proximal severe ischemia and misinterpreted as a consequence of stroke. Usually paralysis is more obscure, however, presenting as a decreased strength and mobility in the most distal parts of the leg where the ischemia is most severe. The most sensitive test of motor function is to ask the patient to try to move and spread the toes. This gives information about muscular function in the foot and calf. Bending the knee joint or lifting the whole leg is accomplished by large muscle groups in the thigh that remain intact for a long time after ischemic damage in the calf muscle and foot has become irreversible.

10.3.3 Evaluation of Severity of Ischemia

10.3.3.1 Classification

When a patient has been diagnosed to have acute leg ischemia, it is extremely important to evaluate its grade. Ischemic severity is the most important factor for selecting a management strategy, and it also affects treatment outcome. Classification according to severity must be done before the patient is moved to the floor or sent to the radiology department. We have found that the simple classification suggested by the Society for Vascular Surgery ad hoc committee (1997) is helpful for grading. It is displayed in Table 10.3.

Table 10.3. Categories of acute ischemia

		Sensibility	Motor function	Arterial Doppler signal	Venous Doppler signal
I	Viable	Normal	Normal	Audible (>30 mmHg)	Audible
IIa	Marginally threatened	Decreased or normal in the toes	Normal	Not audible	Audible
IIb	Immediately threatened	Decreased, not only in the toes	Mildly to moderately affected	Not audible	Audible
IV	Irreversibly damaged	Extensive anesthesia	Paralysis and rigor	Not audible	Not audible

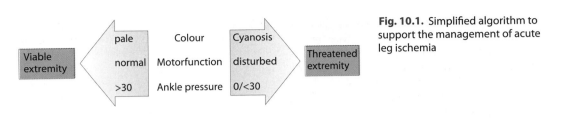

Fig. 10.1. Simplified algorithm to support the management of acute leg ischemia

10.3.3.2 Viable Leg

As indicated in Figure 10.1, a viable ischemic leg is not cyanotic, the toes can be moved voluntarily, and the ankle pressure is measurable. The rationale for choosing these parameters is that cyanosis and impaired motor function are of high prognostic value for outcome.

The limit of 30 mmHg for the ankle pressure (Table 10.3, Fig. 10.1) is not important per se but is a practical limit useful to make sure that it is the arterial, and not a venous, pressure that has been measured. The dorsalis pedis, posterior tibial arteries, or branches from the peroneal artery can be insonated. The latter can be found just ventral to the lateral malleolus. If no audible signal is identified in any of these arteries or if there only is a weak signal that disappears immediately when the tourniquet is inflated, the ankle blood pressure should be recorded as zero. It is important to rely on the obtained results and not assume that there is a signal somewhere that is missed due to inexperience. Qualitative analysis of the Doppler signal is seldom useful when evaluating acute leg ischemia.

10.3.3.3 Threatened Leg

As shown in Table 10.3, the threatened leg differs from the viable one in that the sensibility is impaired and there is no measurable ankle blood pressure. The threatened limb is further separated into marginally threatened and immediately threatened by the presence or absence of normal motor function. The threatened leg differs from the irreversibly damaged leg by the quality of the venous Doppler signal. In the irreversibly damaged leg, venous blood flow is stagnant and inaudible.

10.3.3.4 Management Strategy

A viable leg does not require immediate action and can be observed in the ward. A threatened leg needs urgent operation or thrombolysis. The latter is more time-consuming and recommended for the marginally threatened leg. The immediately threatened leg must be treated as soon as possible, usually with embolectomy or a vascular reconstruction. Irreversible ischemia is quite unusual but implies that the patient's leg cannot be saved. Figure 10.1 is intended to show a simplified algorithm to further support the management of acute leg ischemia.

NOTE

Loss of motor function in the calf and foot muscles warrants emergency surgical treatment.

10.4 Diagnostics

A well-conducted physical examination is enough to confirm the diagnosis of acute leg ischemia, determine the level of obstruction, and evaluate the severity of ischemia. When the leg is immediately threatened, further radiologic examinations or vascular laboratory tests should not under any circumstances delay surgical treatment. When the extremity is viable or marginally threatened, angiography should be performed. Duplex ultrasound is of limited value for evaluating acute leg ischemia and angiography is recommended for almost all patients in these two groups. If angiography is not available or if examination of the patient has verified that emboli is the cause and probably is best treated by embolectomy, angiography can be omitted. This situation is rare, however.

The arteriogram provides an anatomical map of the vascular bed and is very helpful in discriminating embolus and thrombosis. The former is essential for planning the surgical procedure, and the latter may be of importance for selecting the treatment strategy.

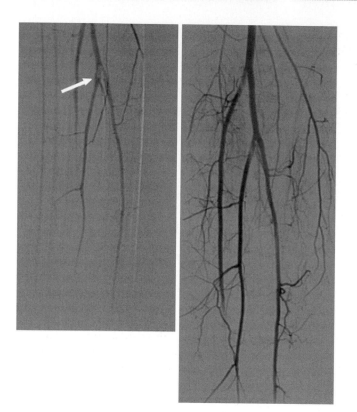

An arteriogram representing an embolus is shown in Fig. 10.2.

Angiographic signs of embolism are an abrupt, convex start of the occlusion and lack of collaterals. Thrombosis is likely when the arteriogram shows well-developed collaterals and atherosclerotic changes in other vascular segments.

For most patients with viable and marginally threatened legs the diagnostic angiography is followed by therapeutic thrombolysis right away.

Angiography can be performed during daytime when qualified radiology staff is available. The patient should be optimized according to the recommendations given in the next section. Before angiography it is important to keep the patient well hydrated and to stop administration of metformin to reduce the risk of renal failure. Disturbances in coagulation parameters may interfere with arterial puncture and must also be checked before the investigation. The information is also important as baseline values in case of later thrombolysis.

The groin of the contralateral leg is the preferred puncture site for diagnostic angiography. A second antegrade puncture can be done in the ischemic extremity if thrombolysis is feasible.

10.5 Management and Treatment

10.5.1 Management Before Treatment

10.5.1.1 Viable Leg

If the leg is viable the patient is admitted for observation. A checklist of what needs to be done in the emergency department follows below:

1. Place an intravenous (IV) line.
2. Start infusion of fluids. Because dehydration is often a part of the pathogenic process, Ringer's acetate is usually preferred. Dextran is another option that also is beneficial for blood rheology.
3. Draw blood for hemoglobin and hematocrit, prothrombin time, partial thromboplastin time, complete blood count, creatinine, blood

urea nitrogen, fibrinogen, and antithrombin. Consider the need to type and cross-match blood.

4. Order an electrocardiogram (ECG).
5. Administer analgesics according to pain intensity. Opiates are usually required (morphine 2.5–10 mg IV).
6. Consider heparinization, especially if only Ringer's acetate is given. Heparin treatment should be postponed until after surgery if epidural anesthesia is likely.

Repeated assessments of the patient's clinical status are mandatory in the intensive care unit and when the patient has been moved to the ward. The time interval depends on the severity of ischemia and the medical history. This examination includes evaluating skin color, sensibility, and motor function as well as asking the patient about pain intensity.

Dextran is administered throughout the observation period. The risk for deterioration of heart failure due to dextran treatment is substantial and for patients at risk the volume load must be related to the treatment's expected possible benefits. For such patients it is wise to reduce the normal dose of 500 ml in 12 h to 250 ml. Another option is to prolong the infusion time to 24 h.

Heparin only or in combination with dextran is recommended when patients do have an embolic source or a coagulation disorder. There are two ways to administer heparin. The first is the standard method, consisting of a bolus dose of 5,000 units IV followed by infusion of heparin solution (100 units/ml) with a drop counter. The dose at the start of infusion should be 500 units of heparin per kilogram of body weight per 24 h. The dose is then adjusted according to activated partial thromboplastin time (APTT) values obtained every 4 h. The APTT value should be 2–2.5 times the baseline value.

Low molecular weight heparin administered subcutaneously twice daily is the other option. A common dose is 10,000 units/day but it should be adjusted according to the patient's weight.

It is important to optimize cardiac and pulmonary function while monitoring the patient. Hypoxemia, anemia, arrhythmia, and hypotension worsen ischemia and should be abolished if possible. A cardiology consult is often needed.

The above-mentioned treatment regime of rehydration, anticoagulation, and optimization of cardiopulmonary function often improves the ischemic leg substantially. Frequently this is enough to sufficiently restore perfusion in the viable ischemic leg, and no other treatments are needed. If no improvement occurs, angiography can be performed during the daytime, followed by thrombolysis, PTA, or vascular reconstruction.

10.5.1.2 Threatened Leg

If the leg is immediately threatened, the patient is prepared for operation right away. This includes the steps listed above for the viable leg, including contact with an anesthesiologist. When there is no cyanosis and motor function is normal – that is, the extremity is only marginally threatened – there is time for immediate angiography followed by thrombolysis or operation. An option is cautious monitoring and angiography as soon as possible.

Before starting the operation, the surgeon needs to consider the risk for having to perform a complete vascular reconstruction. It is probable that a bypass to the popliteal artery or a calf artery will be needed to restore circulation. If thrombosis is the likely cause and the obstruction is distal (a palpable pulse is felt in the groin but not distally), a bypass may also be required even when embolization is suspected.

10.5.2 Operation

10.5.2.1 Embolectomy

It is beyond the scope of this book to cover the technique for vascular reconstructions. But because embolectomy from the groin with balloon catheters (known as Fogarty catheters) is one of the most common emergency vascular operations in a general surgical clinic and may be performed by surgeons not so familiar with vascular surgery, this is described in the Technical Tips box below.

TECHNICAL TIPS
Embolectomy

Use an operating table that allows x-ray penetration. Local anesthesia is used if embolus is likely and the obstruction seems to be in the upper thigh or in pelvic vessels (no pulse in the groin). Make a longitudinal incision in the skin, and identify and expose the common, superficial, and deep femoral arteries (Chapter 9, p. 107). If the common femoral artery is soft-walled and free from arteriosclerosis – especially if a pounding pulse is felt proximal to the origin of the deep femoral artery – an embolus located in its bifurcation is likely. Make a short transverse arteriotomy including almost half the circumference. Place the arteriotomy only a few mm proximal to the origin of the profunda artery so it can be inspected and cannulated with ease. In most other cases, a longitudinal arteriotomy is preferable because it allows elongation and can be used as the site for the inflow anastomosis of a bypass. For proximal embolectomy, a #5 catheter is used.

Before the catheter is used the balloon should be checked by insufflation of a suitable volume of saline. Check the position of the lever of the syringe when the balloon is starting to fill, which gives a good idea of what is happening inside the artery. Wet the connection piece for the syringe to get a tight connection. It is smart to get external markers of the relationship between the catheter length and important anatomical structures; for example, the aortic bifurcation (located at the umbilicus level), the trifurcation level (located approximately 10 cm below the knee joint), as well as the ankle level. The catheters have centimeter grading, which simplifies the orientation.

It is common for the embolus to already be protruding when the arteriotomy is done and a single pull with the catheter starting with the tip in the iliac artery is enough to ensure adequate inflow. This means that a strong pulse can be found above the arteriotomy, and a pulsatile heavy blood flow comes through the nole. For distal clot extraction, a #3 or #4 catheter is recommended. A slight bending of the catheter tip between the thumb and index finger might, in combination with rotation of the catheter, make it easier to pass down the different arterial branches (Fig. 10.3).

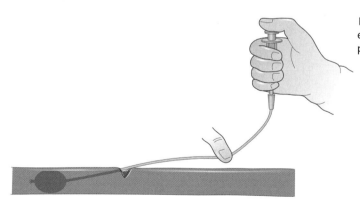

Fig. 10.3. Use of Fogarty catheter for embolectomy. Note that withdrawal is parallel to the artery

When the catheter is inserted into the artery and while the surgeon is working with it, hemostasis of the arteriotomy is achieved by a vessel-loop or by a thumb–index finger grip over the artery and the catheter. In a typical case, an embolus, including a possible secondary thrombus, can be passed relatively easily or with only slight resistance. If a major part of the catheter can be inserted the tip will be located in one of the calf arteries, most probably the posterior tibial artery or the peroneal artery. The balloon is insufflated simultaneously as the catheter is slowly withdrawn, which makes it easier to get a feeling for the dynamics and to not apply too much pressure against the vascular wall. A feeling of "touch" is preferable, but a feeling of "pull" against the vascular wall should be avoided.

To get the right feeling the same person needs to hold the catheter, pull it, and insufflate the balloon at the same time. To avoid damage in the arteriotomy, the direction of withdrawal should be parallel with the artery (Fig. 10.3).

When the catheter is withdrawn it moves into larger segments of the artery and has to be successively insufflated until it reaches the arteriotomy. The reverse is, of course, valid when the embolectomy is done in a proximal direction. The thromboembolic masses can be suctioned or pulled out with forceps, and the arteriotomy should be inspected to be clean from remaining materials before the catheter is reinserted. The maneuver should be repeated until the catheter has been passed at least once without any exchange of thromboembolic materials and until there is an acceptable backflow from the distal vascular bed. Depending on the degree of ischemia and collaterals, the backflow is, however, not always brisk.

If a catheter runs into early and hard resistance, this might be due to previously occluded segment that forced the catheter into a branch. It should then be withdrawn and reinserted, using great caution to avoid perforation. If the resistance cannot be passed and if acute ischemia is present, angiography should always be considered to examine the possibility of a vascular reconstruction.

Besides performing embolectomy in the superficial femoral, popliteal, and calf arteries, the deep femoral artery must be checked for an obstructing embolus or clot that needs to be extracted. Separate declamping of the superficial femoral and deep femoral arteries to check the backflow is the best way to do this. Remember the possibility that backflow from the distal vascular bed after embolectomy might emanate from collaterals located proximal to distally located clots. Back flow does not always assure that the peripheral vascular bed is free from further embolic masses. A basic rule is that every operation should be completed with intraoperative angiography (see the technical tips box in the next page and Fig. 10.4) to ensure good outflow and to rule out remaining emboli and secondary thrombus. To dissolve small amounts of remaining thrombus local infusion of 2–4 cc recombinant tissue plasminogen activator (rtPA) can be administered before the angiography catheter is pulled out.

Finally, the arteriotomy is closed. If necessary a patch of vein or synthetic material is used to avoid narrowing of the lumen.

As mentioned before, the embolectomy procedure includes intraoperative angiography. If this examination indicates significant amounts of emboli remaining in the embolectomized arteries or if the foot still appears as being inadequately perfused after the arteriotomy is closed, other measures need to be taken. If there are remaining emboli in the superficial femoral or popliteal arteries, another embolectomy attempt from the arteriotomy in the groin can be made. Clots, if seen in all the calf arteries, need to be removed through a second arteriotomy in the popliteal artery. This is done by a medial incision below the knee; note that local anesthesia is not sufficient for this. It is usually necessary to restore flow in two, or occasionally in only one, of the calf arteries.

Embolectomy at the popliteal level is the first treatment step when ischemia is limited to the distal calf and foot and when there is a palpable pulse in the groin or in the popliteal fossa.

NOTE

Do not forget to consider fasciotomy in patients with severe ischemia.

◼ 10.5.2.2 Thrombosis

The preliminary diagnosis of embolus must be reconsidered if the exposed femoral artery in the groin is hard and calcified. In most situations, clot removal with Fogarty catheters will then fail. It is usually difficult or even impossible to pass the catheter distally, indicating the presence of stenoses or occlusions. Even if the embolectomy appears successful, early reocclusion is common. Such secondary thrombosis is usually more extensive and will aggravate the ischemia. Accordingly, angiography should be considered as the first step if the femoral artery is grossly arteriosclerotic and if it is hard to pass the catheter down to the calf level. It will confirm the etiology and reveal whether a bypass is required and feasible. Vascular reconstruction in acute leg ischemia is often rather difficult and experience in vascular surgery is required.

10.5.2.3 Intraoperative angiography

> **TECHNICAL TIPS**
> **Intraoperative angiography**
>
> With the proximal clamp in position a 5 or 8 French baby-feeding catheter is inserted into the arteriotomy. The tip of the catheter is placed 5 cm into the superficial femoral artery and distal control around it is achieved with a vessel-loop. Contrast for intravasal use containing 140–300 mg iodine/ml is infused with a 20 cc syringe connected to a three-way valve. Heparinized Ringer's or saline (10 units/ml heparin) is flushed through the catheter before and after contrast injection to prevent thrombosis in the occluded vascular bed.
>
> If the patient is suspected to have renal failure, the amount of contrast used is kept at a minimum. Angled projections can be obtained without moving the C-arm by rotating the patient's foot. The use of contrast in the Fogarty catheter balloon during fluoroscopy allows the calf vessel into which the catheter slides to be identified. The technique for intraoperative angiography is also a prerequisite for interoperative use of endovascular treatment options such as angioplasty (Fig. 10.4).

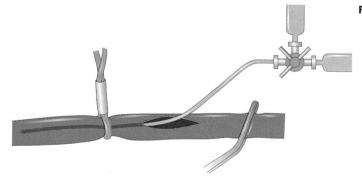

Fig. 10.4. Intraoperative angiography

10.5.3 Thrombolysis

Thrombolysis is performed in the angiosuite. A consultation with a specialist in coagulation disorders or a specialist in vascular medicine is sometimes needed to discuss possible problems related to coagulation before the procedure. Contraindications to thrombolysis are listed in Table 10.4.

Treatment is usually directed toward resolving a fresh, thrombotic occlusion, but emboli and thrombi several weeks old can also be successfully lysed. The procedure starts with a diagnostic angiography via contralateral or antegrade ipsilateral arterial punctures. If thrombolytic treatment is decided the procedure continues right away, and the tip of a pulse-spray catheter is placed in the thrombus. The lytic agent is then forcefully injected directly into it to cause fragmentation. The primary choices for lytic agent are recombinant tissue plasminogen activator (rtPA) or urokinase. Because of the risk of allergic reactions, streptokinase should be avoided. Intermittent injections of

Table 10.4. Some contraindications to thrombolysis

Absolute	Relative
Cerebrovascular incident <2 months	Major surgery or trauma <10 days
Active bleeding diathesis	Uncontrolled hypertension (>180 systolic)
Gastrointestinal bleeding <10 days	Hepatic failure
	Pregnancy
	Severe renal failure
	Diabetic retinopathy

1 ml every 5–10 min to a total dose of 10–20 ml rtPA over 1–3 h is followed by angiographic control of the result. If the thrombus is completely lysed any underlying lesion is treated. If thrombus still remains, the rtPA infusion is continued slowly over 6–12 h with 1 mg/h. If the initial thrombolysis fails, a variety of mechanical catheters can be used to try to further dissolve and aspirate the thrombus. Examples include the AngioJet and the Amplatz.

Because of the risk of bleeding and systemic complications, and also because the ischemic leg may deteriorate, careful monitoring during continued thrombolysis is necessary. This is best done in an intensive care or step-down unit. The patient should be kept supine in bed throughout the procedure. During this time the other measures suggested for optimizing coagulation and central circulation are continued. It is also necessary to check fibrinogen concentration to make sure the value does not decline to <1.0 mg/ml. Below this level surgical hemostasis is insufficient and the infusion should be stopped. Angiographic control of the result is performed afterwards, usually the following morning, and occasionally during the slow infusion to check the effect and allow repositioning of the catheter. The part of the thrombus surrounding the catheter is lysed first, which is why it often is beneficial to advance the catheter further into the thrombus after a few hours.

Finally, the lesion that caused the thrombosis is treated with angioplasty. To avoid unnecessary bleeding from the puncture site, the fibrinogen concentration is checked again before the sheath is withdrawn to ensure that the level exceeds 1.0 mg/ml.

10.5.4 Management After Treatment

10.5.4.1 Anticoagulation

Patients with embolic disease caused by cardiac arrhythmia or from other cardiac sources proven by ECG, medical history, or clinical signs should be anticoagulated postoperatively. Treatment regimens described previously (page 125) are employed, followed by treatment with coumadin. Anticoagulation has no proven positive effect for the prognosis of the ischemic leg but is administered to reduce the risk of new emboli. The patient's abilities to comply with treatment and the risk for bleeding complications have to be weighed against the benefits. If the source of the emboli is not clear, it should be investigated. Findings of atrial fibrillation and heart thrombus can then be treated. If the ECG is normal, echocardiography is ordered to search for thrombus and valve deficiencies. If the left atrium is a likely embolic source, transesophageal echocardiography may be indicated.

When the etiology of leg ischemia is uncertain it is difficult to give general advice. There is no scientific evidence that long-term postoperative anticoagulation reduces the risk of reocclusion or influences patient survival. Continued treatment with dextran or low molecular weight heparin is recommended at least during hospitalization.

If hypercoagulable states are suspected the patient needs to be worked up during the postoperative period to reduce the risk of reocclusion. Examples are patients with hyperhomocysteinemia, who may be treated with folates, and patients with antiphospholipid antibodies, who need coumadin and salicylic acid.

10.5.4.2 Reperfusion Syndrome

Patients treated for severe acute leg ischemia are at risk of developing reperfusion syndrome. This occurs when ischemic muscles are reperfused and metabolites from damaged and disintegrated muscle cells are spread systemically. A part of this process consists of leakage of myoglobin; it may be nephrotoxic and colors the urine red. The metabolites also affect central circulation and may cause arrhythmia and heart failure. The risk for reperfusion syndrome is higher when occlusions are proximal and the affected muscle mass is large. One example is saddle emboli located in the iliac bifurcation. The risk is also higher when the ischemia time is longer than 4–6 h.

The elevated mortality associated with severe acute leg ischemia may be due to reperfusion syndrome. Survival may therefore be improved by avoiding reperfusion and a lower mortality has been reported from hospitals where primary amputation is favored. It has also been suggested that thrombolysis saves lives by restoring perfusion gradually. For a threatened leg this is seldom an option because rapid restoration of perfusion is necessary to save it.

The best treatment for reperfusion syndrome is prevention by expeditious restoration of flow.

There are no clinically proven effective drugs but many have been successful in animal models, including heparin, mannitol, and prostaglandins. Because heparin and mannitol also have other potential benefits and few side effects they are recommended during the postoperative period. Obviously, acidosis and hyperkalemia must be corrected, and the patient needs to be well hydrated and have good urine output.

For patients with suspected reperfusion syndrome – urine acidosis and high serum myoglobin levels – alkalinization of the urine is often recommended in order to avoid renal failure despite weak support in the literature. If the urine is red, the urine pH <7.0, and serum myoglobin >10,000 mg/ml, 100 ml sodium bicarbonate is given IV. The dose is repeated until the pH is normalized.

10.5.4.3 Compartment Syndrome

The acute inflammation in the muscle after reestablishing perfusion leads to swelling and a risk for compartment syndrome. The available space for the muscles is limited in the leg and when the increased pressure in the compartments reduces capillary perfusion below the level necessary for tissue viability, nerve injury and muscle necrosis occur.

The essential clinical feature of compartment syndrome is pain – often very strong and "out of proportion," which is accentuated by passive extension. The muscle is hard and tender when palpated. Unfortunately, nerves within the compartments are also affected, causing disturbance of sensibility and motor function. This makes diagnosis more difficult. Moreover, the patient is often not fully awake or disoriented, but early diagnosis is still important to save the muscle tissue. For that reason measurement of intracompartmental pressure is performed for diagnosis in some hospitals. There are no precise limits that advocate fasciotomy, but 30 mmHg has been proposed. The specificity for a correct diagnosis using this limit is high, but the sensitivity is much lower.

To notice signs of compartment syndrome after operation or thrombolysis for acute ischemia, frequent physical examinations are vital. Fasciotomy should be performed immediately following the procedure if any suspicion of compartment syndrome exists. Common advice is to always perform fasciotomy right after the vascular procedure when the ischemia is severe and has lasted over 4–6 h. To open all four compartments, we recommend using two long incisions, one placed laterally and one medially in the calf. The technique is described and illustrated in Chapter 9 (p. 115–116).

10.6 Results and Outcome

The outlook for patients with acute leg ischemia has generally been poor. The 30-day mortality when an embolus is the etiology varies between 10% and 40%. Survival is better when arterial thrombosis is the cause, around 90%. When considering the amputation rate after surgical treatment the figures are reversed – lower for embolic disease, at 10–30%, than for thrombosis, which often has an early amputation rate of around 40%.

A substantial number of the patients die or require amputation after 30 days. This is due to a combined effect of the patients' advanced age and comorbidities. In studies not differentiating between etiologies, only 30–40% of the patients were alive 5 years after surgery, and among those, 40–50% had had amputations.

Because the gradual release of ischemia is thought to reduce the risk for reperfusion syndrome and thereby the negative effects on the heart and kidneys mortality after thrombolysis is thought to be lower. It is difficult, however, to find data on thrombolytic therapy comparable to surgical results. A majority of patients will undergo surgery when thrombolysis is not technically possible, leaving a selected group to follow up. In the few randomized controlled trials that compare surgery and thrombolysis the short-term and long-term amputation rates are alike. Survival is also similar, but in one study it was lower after thrombolytic therapy at 1 year, 80%, compared with surgically treated patients, of whom only 60% were alive at that time.

10.7 Conditions Associated with Acute Leg Ischemia

10.7.1 Chronic Ischemia of the Lower Extremity

It is sometimes difficult to differentiate between acute leg ischemia, deterioration of chronic leg ischemia, and just severe end-stage chronic disease in general. Periods of pain escalation bring patients with chronic ischemia to the emergency department. Accentuated pain in these patients has a wide range of origins. Decreased foot perfusion can be due to dehydration or lowered systemic pressure as a consequence of heart failure or a change in medication. Ulcers are frequently painful, especially when complicated by infection or when dressings are changed. History and examination of vital functions and the leg usually disclose such conditions and can also sufficiently rule out acute leg ischemia that needs urgent treatment.

Patients with chronic ischemia benefit from careful planning of their treatment and should not – with few exceptions – be expeditiously treated. Elective therapy includes weighing risk factors against the outcome of the proposed treatment and all the work-up that is needed to get this information. (It is beyond this book's purpose to describe the management of chronic ischemia.) In the emergency department it is sensible to identify and directly treat the patients with true acute leg ischemia and schedule treatment of patients with chronic disease for later. Examples of findings in medical history and physical examination are listed in Table 10.5

Table 10.5. Medical history and physical examination findings suggesting chronic leg ischemia

History	Examination
Coronary artery disease and stroke	Lack of palpable pulses in both legs
Smoking	Ankle pressure 15–50 mmHg
Claudication, rest pain, and ischemic ulcers	Ulcers
Previous vascular surgery or amputation	Hyperemic foot skin while dependent
Lack of sudden onset of pain	

10.7.2 Acute Ischemia After Previous Vascular Reconstruction

A substantial number of patients have chronic leg ischemia and have undergone vascular reconstructions, so there is a high likelihood that emergency department physicians will have to take care of problems with postoperative acute leg ischemia in the operated leg. The clinical presentation of graft failure or occlusion is variable. An abrupt change in leg function and skin temperature accompanied by the onset of pain can occur any time after surgery, but especially within the first 6 months. Several years after the reconstruction it is slightly more common for progressive deterioration to occur and an eventual graft occlusion to pass unnoticed.

As discussed previously in this chapter the management principles are roughly the same as for primary acute leg ischemia. It is the status of the leg and the severity of ischemia that lead work-up and management. Most patients will undergo angiography to establish diagnosis and to provide information about possibilities to restore blood flow. Thrombolysis is often the best treatment option because it exposes the underlying lesions that may have caused the occlusion. As for patients with acute ischemia, those with an immediately threatened leg after a reconstruction should be taken to the operating room and treated as fast as possible. Management of acute ischemia after a previous vascular reconstruction is further discussed in Chapter 12 on complications in vascular surgery.

10.7.3 Blue Toe Syndrome

A toe that suddenly becomes cool, painful, and cyanotic, while pulses can be palpated in the foot, characterizes the classic presentation of blue toe syndrome. This has occasionally led to the assumption that the discoloration of the toe is not of vascular origin, and patients have been sent home without proper vascular assessment. Although coagulation disorders or vasculitis may contribute, such an assumption is dangerous. Atheroembolism is the main cause for blue toe syndrome and atheromatous plaques in the iliac or femoral arteries or thrombi in abdominal or popliteal aneurysms are the main sources. Blue toe syndrome can also present without palpable foot pulses. The presentation may then be less dramatic.

It is common that the patient does not notice the initial insult and wait to seek medical care until after several weeks. Ischemic ulceration at the tip of the toe may then be found in the examination. During the foot examination more signs of microembolization are usually found, including blue spots or patchy discoloration of the sole and heel. When both feet are affected it suggests an embolic source above the aortic bifurcation. The clinical examination should include assessing the aorta and all peripheral arteries, including pulses and auscultation for bruits. When pulses in the foot are not palpable, ankle blood pressure needs to be measured. In the search for aneurysms and stenoses patients need to be investigated with duplex ultrasound to verify examination findings. To prevent future embolization episodes lesions or aneurysms found should be treated as soon as possible.

Occasionally the pain is transient and the blue color will disappear within a few weeks. More common, however, is an extremely intense pain in the toe that is continuous and difficult to treat. Unfortunately, the pain often lasts several months until the toe is either amputated or healed.

The pain is best treated with oral opiates, and quite high doses are often required to ease the pain. A tricyclic antidepressant drug may be added to the regimen if analgesics are not enough.

While waiting for diagnostic studies and final treatment of the lesions, the patient is put on aspirin therapy. There is no scientific evidence for using other medications such as coumadin, steroids, or dipyramidole. Still, if suspicion for a popliteal aneurysm is high we recommend anticoagulation with low molecular weight heparin until the aneurysm is corrected.

10.7.4 Popliteal Aneurysms

A common reason for acute leg ischemia is thrombosis of a popliteal aneurysm. Such aneurysms are also one of the main sources for embolization to the digits in the foot and blue toe syndrome. Besides the clinical signs of acute ischemia discussed previously, a prominent wide popliteal pulse or a mass in the popliteal fossa is often palpated when popliteal aneurysm is the reason for the obstruction.

Popliteal aneurysms are frequent in men but rare in women. They are often bilateral – more than 50% – and associated with the presence of other aneurysms. For instance, 40% of patients with popliteal aneurysms also have an aneurysm in the abdominal aorta.

Most popliteal aneurysms are identified during angiography performed as part of the management process for acute leg ischemia. When an aneurysm is suspected during angiography or examination, duplex ultrasound is performed to verify the finding and estimate the aneurysm's diameter.

If the severity of ischemia corresponds to the "immediately threatened" stage described earlier, the patient needs urgent surgery. The revascularization procedure is then often quite difficult. Exposure of the popliteal artery below the knee, including the origins of the calf arteries, should be followed by intraoperative angiography and an attempt to remove the thrombus. It is hoped that angiography can identify a spared calf artery distally. The calf arteries are sometimes slightly dilated in this patient group and can serve as a good distal landing site for a bypass excluding the aneurysm. Often, however, it is impossible to open up the distal vascular bed due to old embolic occlusions and the prognosis for the leg is poor. In such situations every possible alternative solution should be considered, including local thrombolysis, systemic prostaglandin infusion, and profundaplasty.

If the ischemia is less severe, thrombolysis may be considered following the angiography before surgical exclusion of the aneurysm. While thrombolysis previously has been considered questionable because of the risk for further fragmentation of thrombus within the popliteal aneurysm, this strategy may prove very favorable. Over the last few years several studies reporting restored calf vessels by thrombolysis have been published. This may lead to more successful bypasses and improved limb salvage. Once the bypass is accomplished good long-term results are probable. Interestingly, vein grafts used for bypasses in patients with popliteal aneurysms appear to be wider and stay patent longer than for other patient groups.

Further Reading

Berridge DC, Kessel D, Robertson I. Surgery versus thrombolysis for acute limb ischaemia: initial management. Cochrane Database Syst Rev 2002; (3): CD002784

Dormandy J, Heeck L, Vig S. Acute limb ischemia. Semin Vasc Surg 1999; 12(2):148153

Henke PK, Stanley JC. The treatment of acute embolic lower limb ischemia. Adv Surg 2004; 38:281–291

Galland RB. Popliteal aneurysms: controversies in their management. Am J Surg 2005; 190(2):314–318

O'Donnell TF Jr. Arterial diagnosis and management of acute thrombosis of the lower extremity. Can J Surg 1993; 36(4):349–353

Ouriel K. Endovascular techniques in the treatment of acute limb ischemia: thrombolytic agents, trials, and percutaneous mechanical thrombectomy techniques. Semin Vasc Surg 2003; 16(4):270–279

General Concepts

PART B

Vascular Access in Trauma   11

CONTENTS

11.1 Summary

- Make sure you are familiar with the tech niques for vascular access before the trau ma case arrives.
- Use the technique for vascular access in which you are most experienced.
- Do not hesitate to start simultaneous expo sure of several different veins.
- Do not forget the cubital fossa as a possible site for vein exposure.

11.2 Background

Optimal management of a trauma case includes fast resuscitation, diagnosis, and immediate start of treatment. In most injured patients, two large peripheral intravenous (IV) lines are sufficient to provide adequate initial treatment and volume replacement. In rare cases of greater trauma and in unclear cases this might be insufficient and sev eral (sometimes central) IV lines are needed. In bleeding shock with collapsed and empty veins, inserting peripheral IV lines are difficult. For these reasons some techniques for alternative ac cess should be included in the armamentarium of all physicians who take part in the management of trauma cases. In many hospitals the general sur geon on call is in charge of the trauma care and is thus responsible for providing adequate vascular access.

11.3 Management

11.3.1 In the Emergency Department

Today most trauma patients admitted to emergen cy departments already have one or two peripheral IV cannulas that were inserted by the paramed ics.

After securing airways and respiration, the sur geon on call checks the patient for possible ongo ing and previous bleeding and estimates the blood losses. Besides being part of trauma management, this information is also necessary for planning the need for vascular access. According to our rou tines all trauma cases are subjected to immediate infusion of 2 l of Ringer's acetate. If this volume has a positive effect on tachycardia and the pa tient's general condition, and the patient is not ob viously bleeding externally, the total possible blood loss will usually not exceed 15–20% of the total blood volume. For these patients two large-bore IV cannulas (2 mm in diameter) are almost always enough for the initial volume replacement. The order in which the volume replacement should be done and in what proportion the Ringer's, blood, plasma, packed cells, or dextran should be given varies between hospitals and should, of course, be in accordance with local prescriptions and routines.

11.3.1.1 Management Guidelines in Acute Vascular Access

Always start by checking that the patient has two functioning IV cannulas. If they are functioning but are too small in caliber – <1 mm in diameter – a guide wire can be used to replace them with larger ones. Insert the guide wire in the thin cannula, pull it out over the guide wire, leave the guide wire in the vein, and insert a new wider IV cannula over the guide wire. Occasionally the skin perforation is too small and needs to be dilated. The cannula replacement should be performed simultaneously with another person's attempt to place IV cannulas in other sites. Patients with greater ongoing bleeding, such as a patient who is bleeding through a fresh wound dressing within a minute, as well as those with a history that indicates larger blood losses, almost uniformly require several IV cannulas. Short and large-bore cannulas permit the highest possible volume flow and if there is space available on the arms and neck more peripheral cannulas are warranted. Make simultaneous attempts at several different sites – for example, in the external jugular vein and in the veins on the hands. If this is not successful there are three alternatives:

1. Surgical exposure of veins in the cubital fossa or on the leg
2. Percutaneous catheterization of the femoral vein
3. Central venous catheterization in the subclavian vein or external and internal jugular vein

The best choice of these three alternatives is not always obvious and should be based on factors such as the part of the patient's body that is injured, the responsible trauma surgeon's experience, the urgency and the type of fluid that needs to be infused. The following general advice might be helpful irrespective of the technique chosen:

■ Never place an IV cannula in extremities injured by crush or burn.
■ Avoid extremities with fractures.
■ If larger vascular injuries are suspected, including pelvic fractures, which are frequently associated with extensive venous damage in the pelvis, IV lines should be placed above as well as below the diaphragm to ensure that administered fluid reaches the central circulation and is not lost on the way because of vascular injuries.

Another possibility for acute access is an interosseous cannula. This, however, is not described in this chapter.

11.3.1.2 Which Route is Recommended for Acute Vascular Access?

Some 20 years ago surgical cutdown was the method of choice in trauma because most surgeons used this method electively. At that time it was routine and surgeons could generally insert and fixate a large-bore IV line within just a couple of minutes. Today this experience is generally lacking and trauma care according to Advanced Trauma Life Support, for example, recommends the second alternative listed above, catheterization of the femoral vein. The reason is probably that catheterization of the femoral vein is technically easier to perform for someone surgically inexperienced than surgical cutdown or central catheterization. In many countries, including the United States, catheterization of the jugular and subclavian veins is more widespread, in particular among anesthesiologists.

If cutdown is chosen, most textbooks recommend the greater saphenous vein at the level of the median malleolus as the best, most easily accessible, vein. This technique is identical with the one used in stripping a varicosed greater saphenous vein. The disadvantage is that it is rarely possible to draw blood from the greater saphenous vein at the level of the ankle joint even if the catheter has an intravasal position. This is due to the vein valves and also to the fact that peripheral veins are often collapsed. The patients are frequently in shock as a consequence of severe bleeding. With longer catheters placed in the greater saphenous vein drawing of blood samples is sometimes possible thanks to confluent vein branches. The function is tested by rapid injection of 10–20 cc of saline.

If the patient has pelvic injuries or the best veins have been consumed in previous varicose vein surgery or bypass operations, the cubital fossa is a very good alternative. These veins are also located closer to the heart. In some cases, branches to the greater saphenous in the groin can also be used, especially if the surgeon is experienced in surgical exposures in this area.

11.3.1.3 Technique in Acute Vascular Access

The cutdown technique is described in the Technical Tips box and displayed in Fig. 11.1. Note that the technique is identical to that used for implanting permanent venous infusion ports and other central venous catheters. A surgeon experienced in such procedure can perform a cutdown and catheterization rapidly and effectively. For the same reason, cutdown is probably an underestimated and underused alternative.

Central catheterization is performed in Scandinavia mostly by anesthesiologists and with great skill. This alternative for access in trauma has the disadvantage of long catheters with a relatively small caliber, making rapid infusion of large volumes difficult. Direct puncture in the neck region can be difficult and even dangerous in an anxious and hypoxic patient. In a patient wearing a stiff neck collar it is almost impossible. A central venous catheter allows objective measurement of central venous pressure (CVP), but its value in managing acute trauma is hard to appreciate, and CVP rarely needs to be measured in the emergency situation. The recommendation is therefore to save central catheterization until the most important emergency care is over.

For catheterizing the femoral vein, a Seldinger technique is used. Make sure that suitable sets for catheterization and different catheters are at hand. Previously described problems during cannulation in the lower extremities are, of course, also valid for this technique.

In summary, surgeons managing trauma cases ought to be familiar with one or several different techniques for acute vascular access. This should be practiced beforehand, prior to the arrival of the trauma case in the emergency department.

TECHNICAL TIPS
Vascular Access in Trauma

■ **Technique for exposing the greater saphenous vein[a]**

1. Scrub and drape a 10×10 cm large area anterior to the medial malleolus.
2. If the patient is awake, infiltrate a local anesthetic.
3. Make a 3 cm-long transverse incision anterior to the medial malleolus.
4. Expose the greater saphenous vein by blunt dissection on a length of 2 cm, and protect the saphenous nerve.
5. Pull two absorbable 2-0 sutures under the exposed vein with a clamp.
6. Ligate the vein as far distally as possible with a distal suture. Do not cut the ends of the suture.
7. Place a knot in the proximal suture but do not tie it.
8. Make a transverse cut in the vein with an eye scissor. Do not make it too small. Dilate the venotomy with the tip of a small clamp (mosquito).
9. Insert a catheter a few centimeters while applying slight traction on the distal suture. Tie the proximal suture around the catheter for fixation. If tunnelation is considered, make a second separate incision a few centimeters distally and pull the catheter under the skin before inserting it into the vein (Fig. 11.1).
10. Connect the infusion system and close the wound with a nonresorbable single suture. Do not forget to fix the catheter with a suture to the skin.

---

a) An identical technique can be used to expose and cannulate the cubital vein.

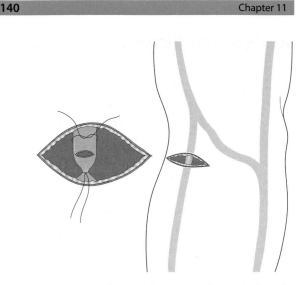

Fig. 11.1. Cutdown and exposure of a vein in the cubital fossa for acute venous access

◼ Further Reading

Klofas E. A quicker saphenous vein cutdown and a better way to teach it. J Trauma 1997; 43:985–987

Waisman M, Waisman D. Bone marrow infusion in adults. J Trauma 1997; 42:288–293

Complications in Vascular Surgery

12

■ 12.1 Summary

- ■ Wound infections may cause life-threatening bleeding by eroding an anastomosis.
- ■ An infected surgical wound overlying a vascular reconstruction should not be debrided in the emergency department.
- ■ A patient with an aortic graft admitted for gastrointestinal bleeding should be treated as having an aortoduodenal fistula.
- ■ Vascular graft infection should be suspected in a patient with unspecific symptoms and a previously implanted aortic graft.
- ■ Leg ischemia following thrombotic occlusion of a previous vascular reconstruction requires careful consideration before a decision to operate, unless the extremity is immediately threatened.
- ■ Suspected extremity or visceral ischemic complications after aortic procedures should be managed in close cooperation with an experienced vascular surgeon.

■ 12.2 Background

The most common complications of vascular surgery – myocardial infarction, aggravated angina, renal insufficiency, and pulmonary problems – will not be dealt with in this chapter. Such systemic complications are consequences of the medical background of vascular surgical patients. In fact, most patients have general manifestations of arteriosclerosis, diabetes, and chronic obstructive pulmonary disease. These risk factors also contribute to the higher incidence of specific complications in this patient group after vascular as well as general surgical procedures. The specific complications of vascular surgical procedures can be categorized into four groups:

1. Ischemic, caused by thrombosis, embolization, dissection, and occlusion of vessels
2. Bleeding
3. Infection in wounds and grafts
4. Local complications in the surgical field.

In this chapter complications will be discussed under headings corresponding to these categories.

■ 12.2.1 Magnitude of the Problem

The number of complications is related to the number of vascular surgical procedures performed. In Sweden, for instance, the number of operations increased from approximately 500 per million inhabitants per year in 1982 to almost 1,200 per million in 1995. A similar pattern is common for most Western countries. The number of procedures, especially endovascular, has continued to rise, and one-third of registered procedures are classified as reoperations. The latter covers revisions of anastomotic problems, angioplasty of restenosis and graft stenosis, operations for acute bleeding, and extirpation of infected grafts.

The incidence of postoperative complications can be estimated from these Swedish data. If approximately 12,000 operations are performed yearly and the risk of complications requiring a visit to the clinic is estimated to be 20%, 2,400 patients will seek medical attention for a complication following a vascular procedure (Table 12.1). In Sweden this corresponds to six or seven patients daily. Most doctors on call will meet such patients and manage their initial work-up and treatment.

■ 12.3 Ischemic Complications

■ 12.3.1 Pathophysiology

Ischemic complications after vascular operations are common and influence several organ systems. Examples of such complications are listed in Table 12.2. There are many different causes and sometimes several factors contribute simultaneously. The consequence is ischemic symptoms in the affected organ.

Vascular reconstructions for chronic leg ischemia have a high risk for developing graft occlusion, especially in the first years after the primary operation. Up to half of the grafts will eventually occlude. The causes for occlusion vary depending on when it occurs. Early (within 30 postoperative days), technical causes dominate, such as a badly sutured anastomosis, intimal tear, and intact valve cusps in an in situ bypass. Other examples are poor vein graft quality and extensive arteriosclerosis in run-off arteries. Late graft occlusion is secondary to intimal hyperplasia in the graft or the

Table 12.1. Frequency of complications after vascular procedures

Category	Type of initial procedure/location	Complication rate of all interventions	Comment
Ischemia	Suprainguinal	15%	Includes endovascular as well as open procedures
	Infrainguinal	20–60%	Graft occlusions only (varies with the level of the distal anastomosis – more distal = higher risk)
	Diagnostic angiography	0.5%	Includes symptomatic embolization
	Aortic surgery	4–5%	Renal insufficiency only (higher risk after operations for rupture)
	Aortic surgery	1%	Intestinal ischemia only after elective surgery (after surgery for rupture, up to 8%)
Bleeding	All types of procedures	1–3%	Bleeding requiring reoperation
Infection	Wound	8–20%	After inguinal incisions with antibiotic prophylaxis
	Aortic graft	1–3%	After surgery for aneurysms as well as occlusive disease
	Femoropopliteal bypass	2–5%	Synthetic grafts only. Considerably lower for vein grafts

Table 12.2. Ischemic complications after vascular interventions (*PTA* percutaneous transluminal angioplasty, *AAA* abdominal aortic aneurysm)

Symptomatic organ	Original procedure	Mechanism	Time when it occurs	Main cause
Leg and foot	Bypass	Graft occlusion	Early and late	Technical errors, intimal hyperplasia
Leg and foot, intestine, kidneys	Aneurysms, PTA	Embolization	Early	Dislodged thrombus
Kidneys	AAA (ruptured)	Clamping, hypovolemia	Early	Impaired renal perfusion
Colon	AAA (ruptured)	Clamping	Early (late)	Ligation of inferior mesenteric artery
Leg and foot, intestine	PTA, all vascular operations	Dissection	Early	Intimal dissection causes vascular occlusion

anastomotic area. Early graft occlusions are generally easier to treat and have a better prognosis.

Embolization and dissection complicates mainly percutaneous transluminal angioplasty (PTA) and angiography. The catheters can dislodge a thrombus located in the abdominal or thoracic aorta that follows the bloodstream to the mesenteric or renal arteries or down into lower extremity vessels. Vigorous manipulation of the aneurysm during surgery for abdominal aortic aneurysms (AAAs) might also cause embolization. This may result in "trash foot," a specific type of acute leg ischemia affecting the foot rather than the entire leg. The name comes from the consequence – that the foot will end up as "trash." It is caused by numerous small emboli occluding distal foot arteries.

Dissection, as a complication of angiography or angioplasty, may also cause ischemia. This might happen anywhere an artery was catheterized, but usually in the aorta. The bloodstream then separates the layers in the vascular wall, creating two separate lumina with blood flow. Most damage occurs when the orifices of the intestinal and renal arteries are occluded by the dissection and these organs become ischemic. This is further described in Chapter 8.

Another type of ischemic complication is multifactorial and follows aortic surgery, usually after emergency operations in which hypovolemic shock is common. Arterial clamping, poor perfusion due to hypovolemia, and hypotension may cause renal failure and ischemic colitis of the sigmoid colon. Reperfusion injury after declamping makes the ischemic consequences worse. Renal insufficiency evolves within 1 week of the operation, but a decrease in urine production is seen immediately after the procedure. Intestinal ischemia usually has an early onset because of postoperative hemodynamic problems but might also be delayed. As soon as the intestinal perfusion is below the critical limit damage will occur.

■ 12.3.2 Clinical Presentation

■ 12.3.2.1 Graft Occlusion in the Leg

Reappearance of preoperative symptoms is the main reason why patients seek help. Often this is worsened claudication, rest pain, or new ulcerations, and the patient describes a sudden onset of symptoms that have deteriorated rapidly. The time of onset coincides with the moment when the graft occludes. It is important to note the time when a venous graft occludes because the endothelium is destroyed within 8–10 h. First appearance of severe problems is regularly preceded by a period of some deterioration, which is caused by a developing stenosis.

It is important to gather as much information as possible about the original operation, the way the graft was tunneled, problems that occurred during the operation (such as poor quality of the vein graft, iatrogenic injuries, problems with inflow), and the result of follow-up examinations. General risk factors also need to be considered if reoperation or thrombolysis is probable.

The physical examination aims to establish the graft occlusion, determining the severity of ischemia and the level of occlusion. This is accomplished by inspecting the foot and leg and by pulse palpation. Furthermore, the ankle-brachial index (ABI) is measured to objectively grade the ischemia. Palpation of pulses along the graft is also helpful to elucidate whether the graft is patent, but interpretation is sometimes difficult. An in situ graft may have pulsations in its proximal parts but be occluded distally with outflow into a residual vein branch. The graft can also be patent despite occlusion of the recipient artery when blood flows in the outflow artery in a retrograde direction. Some grafts are difficult to palpate because they are tunneled deep along the occluded artery. Synthetic grafts are also hard to examine, and a pen Doppler can then identify the graft for palpation. The Doppler signal must also be interpreted with care. The signal may emanate from flow in veins or smaller arteries, so its presence does not guarantee graft patency.

Generally, the medical history and physical examination are sufficient to diagnose the ischemia and if there are no pulses along the graft this suggests occlusion or obstruction. When the examiner is in doubt a duplex examination is performed.

■ 12.3.2.2 Ischemia After Aneurysm Operations and Endovascular Procedures

These complications are discovered in the postoperative period. A patient in the ward who has undergone endovascular treatment and suddenly starts to complain of abdominal pain, a cold painful leg, or more unspecific symptoms should be suspected to be suffering from embolization. The symptoms vary with the vascular segment that has been obstructed. If the superior mesenteric artery is affected, symptoms are similar to those of acute intestinal ischemia (Chapter 6, p. 67). Abdominal pain may also be caused by renal infarction. If a large artery to a lower extremity is occluded, the symptoms are the ones described in Chapter 10 on acute leg ischemia (page 121).

The medical history obtained should include information about the procedure, including whether any problems occurred. For AAA procedures it is important to know if the AAA treated involved the suprarenal or juxtarenal area, if it contained large amounts of thrombus, if it was large, and if it extended into the iliac arteries. The physical examination should cover signs of ischemia and embolization. An example of the latter is skin petechiae in the artery's distribution area. The patient's back and gluteal regions must be examined in addition to the skin of the feet and legs. Patients with "trash foot" or "blue toe syndrome" often have palpable ankle pulses.

After aneurysm operations the patients are often treated in the intensive care unit (ICU) for at least 24 h, and all organ functions are meticulously monitored. After emergency aortic surgery the risk for complications is greater and patients remain in the ICU for several days. Impaired organ perfusion and embolization are common in this group and the nursing staff frequently suspect complications and will alert the doctor on call despite the patient's being under sedation. The primary aim when examining the patient is to diagnose complications requiring immediate surgical treatment, such as intestinal ischemia and large major embolization to the kidneys and legs. Abdominal pain and diarrhea during the first postoperative day, especially if there is blood in the stools, strongly indicates intestinal ischemia. Seventy-five percent of patients with ischemic colitis have diarrhea the first days after surgery. Physical examination findings are a distended abdomen with signs of intestinal paralysis, tenderness in the left lower quadrant, and blood on rectal examination. Patients also have general findings, including fever, acidosis, and oliguria.

Examination of suspected embolization to the legs is more clearcut, with typical findings such as all of the common ones in distal ischemia, as well as absent pulses. Suspicion for renal or intestinal infarction is hard to verify during clinical examination and further investigations with computed tomography (CT) scanning and endoscopy are usually necessary.

12.3.3 Diagnostics

12.3.3.1 Leg Ischemia

No further diagnostic work-up is needed when it is obvious that the patient needs an emergency operation. Examples are immediately threatening leg ischemia and clear vein graft occlusions when thrombolysis not is an alternative. This is the case when more than 72 h have passed since the occlusion occurred or when the patient has recently undergone a surgical or percutaneous procedure. For other patients a duplex examination is the best way to verify graft occlusion as well as occlusion of previously patent native vascular segments in the leg. It is also the first choice in patients with acute complications after endovascular procedures and aortic surgery. Angiography or other radiologic examinations are rarely needed, but they are, of course, required prior to thrombolysis.

12.3.3.2 Visceral Ischemia

Patients with peritonitis and suspected intestinal ischemia do not need work-up and should be taken to the operation room immediately for diagnostic and therapeutic laparotomy. Those with suspected renal or mesenteric artery occlusion, on the other hand, require angiography for an accurate diagnosis. In these segments duplex is obscured by intestinal gas. A very good alternative is CT angiography, which enables identification of renal infarction as well as vascular segments filled with thrombus.

Colon ischemia complicating aortic surgery is sometimes difficult to rule out. The extent of ischemia ranges from a minor mucosal necrosis to transmural intestinal gangrene, and diagnosis is hardest to make early when the changes are minute. Early diagnosis is important to save intestine and to avoid multiple organ failure. The first diagnostic option is coloscopy. Early ischemic signs are a pale mucosa with areas of petechial bleedings. When the mucosa is dark blue or black and partly disintegrated immediate laparotomy is indicated. If a tonometer is available for monitoring mucosal pH in the sigmoid colon it should be placed immediately postoperatively. A pH <7.1 for more than 2 h is considered a strong prognostic sign for the development of intestinal ischemia. The specificity is 90% and the sensitivity 100% if these values are used. A normal CT scan does not exclude ischemic colitis and pathologic CT findings are seen in only one-third of the patients with this diagnosis. Other, but less specific, parameters of possible value are clinical signs of septicemia, increasing lactate concentration in blood, an elevated white blood cell count, and consumption of platelets.

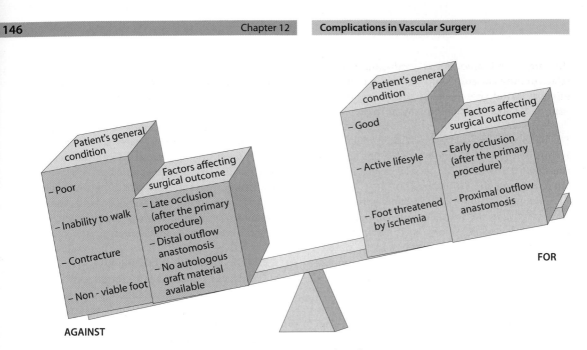

Fig. 12.1. Weighing factors for and against reoperation in graft occlusion

12.3.4 Management and Treatment

12.3.4.1 Management in the Emergency Department, ICU, and the Ward

Leg Ischemia

What previously has been written regarding treatment of acute leg ischemia (Chapter 10) is also valid for leg ischemia as a complication. Patients with an immediately threatened leg – disturbed motor function, no ankle pressure, paralysis – require urgent operation. When a vein graft has occluded treatment should be started as soon as possible even if the leg is not immediately threatened, as the graft can be destroyed within a few hours. It is, however, wise to carefully consider the decision to perform a reoperation. The decision to operate is more difficult than at the primary operation. Necessary information to facilitate the decision includes the reason for occlusion, the indication for the primary operation, risk factors, and available graft material. These factors should be weighed against the expected outcome of the reoperation (Fig. 12.1). For instance, a situation of the initial procedure being leg-saving with an anticipated poor outcome stands against reoperation, as does a bypass to a distal calf artery with a

known poor run-off. A poor general condition of the patient is also a factor that opposes continued active surgical treatment. If the graft occlusion occurred early after the primary operation, thrombectomy alone could possibly be successful.

We prefer to perform angiography as soon as possible regardless of the type of primary operation, duration of graft occlusion, or time of day. Angiography is the first step in thrombolysis and sometimes reveals the reason for the occlusion. If it is impossible for some reason and the leg is threatened, operation is performed right away. The information needed to make a decision to operate or not is obtained from the medical chart, patient interview and physical examination, and angiography findings.

Ischemia After Aneurysm Surgery and Endovascular Procedures

The work-up and treatment for suspected embolization and dissection are difficult but very important because of the fatal consequences that might occur. Patients with postoperative embolization to most arteries in the legs and those with confirmed ischemic colitis and peritonitis, should all be reoperated. The timing depends on the patient's general condition. Frequently it is necessary to optimize the patient medically. When embolization to the intestines is suspected liberal indications for relaparotomy are warranted. For dissections, lowering of blood pressure and endovascular treatment with stents are the first treatments choices.

12.3.4.2 Operation

Embolectomy of the arteries in the legs and intestine has been previously described (Chapters 6 and 10). If examination or angiography indicates that embolizations have occluded distal vessels, clot removal is performed from the popliteal artery or via separate exposure for the tibial arteries. Embolectomy procedures for vascular segments other than those two above require experience from vascular surgery. The surgical treatment of ischemic colitis is usually colon resection (often the sigmoid colon), colostomy, and Hartman closure of the rectum. The difficult part of the operation is to judge whether the colon is ischemic or not. This has also been discussed previously in Chapter 6 and should, of course, comply with prevailing local routines and methods. The principles for thrombolysis are described in Chapter 10. The only surgical procedure that may have to be performed by someone without much experience in vascular surgery is thrombectomy in a vein or synthetic graft; this is briefly described in the Technical Tips box.

TECHNICAL TIPS
Thrombectomy in a Graft

Antibiotic prophylaxis should be given, and the type of anesthesia chosen must allow extensive reconstruction. The distal anastomosis is the most common site for restenosis. A longitudinal incision in the proximal part of the previous incision is used. The advantage with an incision over the anastomosis is that the operation can proceed with revision of the anastomosis if needed. If it has already been decided that the operation is aiming at thrombectomy only, irrespective of the result, the incision is placed where the graft can be palpated easiest. Four to five cm of the graft is exposed first and a vessel loop is applied. A transverse incision is made in the graft without clamping. Thrombectomy is performed with a suitable Fogarty catheter after intravenous (IV)

▼

---

heparin is administered. If acceptable inflow and outflow are accomplished, the graft is occluded with a rubber-covered vascular clamp and the incision is closed with interrupted prolene sutures. If backflow is doubtful and the amount of clot removal is scant, angiography is performed. If the inflow is poor the operation must proceed by exposing the proximal anastomosis. A previously unknown proximal stenosis in the inflow artery or more proximal in the graft is another possible explanation that might require repair. The result of the thrombectomy is controlled either by angiography, continuous-wave Doppler, or palpation.

12.3.4.3 Management After the Operation

Patients who have undergone thrombectomy successfully should receive heparin or low molecular weight heparin according to local protocols. If the reason for graft occlusion is not identified during surgery, the postoperative period is used for workup. Duplex is the first choice for identification of graft problems at this time. In particular, it should look for a stenosed anastomosis or a stenosis in the graft. If thrombosis is unlikely, sources for emboli must be sought. Patients with embolic ischemic complications after aortic surgery or an endovascular procedure who require surgical treatment usually need extensive care in the ICU.

12.3.5 Results and Outcome

12.3.5.1 Graft Occlusion

Results of bypass operations in the legs are usually reported as the share of patent grafts, or the share of salvaged legs, of the total number operated. Accordingly, reoperation or thrombolysis of graft occlusions is so common that it already is considered when results of the primary operation are reported. Outcomes are usually presented as life table curves, where the secondary and sometimes the tertiary patency is reported. The data presented are consequently the number of patent grafts after further treatment with thrombectomy, thrombolysis, and/or revision indicated by graft failure or occlusion, and are defined as secondary patency or primary assisted patency. The difference between primary and secondary patency is, in most reports, 10–15%.

Thrombolysis Versus Thrombectomy

There are no randomized studies of graft occlusion treatment options. It can be assumed that the results of thrombolysis or thrombectomy are similar, providing that the compared groups are stratified according to the cause of graft occlusion. Thrombolysis has the advantage of minimizing the extent of the procedure. In graft occlusion during the immediate postoperative period (2–4 weeks), thrombolysis is associated with an increased risk for bleeding and thrombectomy is safer. Furthermore, several studies report that surgical thrombectomy has the best results when used to treat late occlusions of synthetic grafts, with the distal anastomosis above the knee. Reoperation in theses cases often requires thrombectomy and revision of a stenosed anastomosis with a patch. Above the knee, 52% of the grafts are patent after 3 years and 15% after thrombolysis. The results are better for synthetic grafts compared with vein grafts. It is important, however, to repair the underlying reason for graft occlusion also during thrombolysis. If the reason for occlusion is unknown and not treated, only 10% of grafts are patent 1 year after thrombolytic treatment.

12.3.5.2 Ischemia After AAA Surgery and Endovascular Procedures

Ischemic colitis requiring laparotomy has a 30 day mortality of 50–60% if. If a total colectomy or hemicolectomy was needed the mortality increases to 80%. Interestingly, there doesn't seem to be an increased risk for graft infection after colectomy because of colitis despite the contamination of the abdomen. Extensive embolization to the legs or "trash-foot" after aortic surgery is associated with a 30% mortality within 30 days. Some data in the literature suggest that distal embolectomy from the popliteal or tibial arteries reduces the amputation rate. If the embolization leads to amputation, mortality increases to 40%. Multiple organ failure is associated with an increased risk for all types of complications as well as increased mortality.

12.4 Bleeding Complications

12.4.1 Causes

Bleeding usually happens within 24 h after the primary procedure, but it can occur several years postoperatively. A slipping suture or a leaking anastomosis are the main explanations for perioperative bleedings. Sometimes the condition is accentuated by an increased general tendency for bleeding or by ongoing anticoagulation treatment. Problems with ligatures on vein branches of an in situ infrainguinal vein graft are relatively common. Such ligatures have to resist much stronger forces than normal vein pressure. Late bleeding is caused by infectious erosion of the vascular wall or an anastomosis.

The patient often bleeds considerably before and during acute vascular operations. This results in increased fibrinolysis and consumption of coagulation factors, which may lead to secondary hemostasis problems. Prolonged bleeding time as a consequence of antiplatelet medication is also common. A previously undetected hemophilia can, of course, also cause postoperative hemorrhage, as can overly generous perioperative anticoagulation.

12.4.2 Clinical Presentation

The presentation of bleeding is usually obvious.

12.4.2.1 Medical History

An important part of the medical history is found in the operation note. It describes technical difficulties, iatrogenic vascular injuries, and other problems. Information about preoperative bleeding, substitution, and systemic anticoagulation is found in anesthesia notes. A history of a previous tendency to bleed (for instance, difficulties stopping bleeding after minor wounds, a tendency to bruise easily, or bleeding during tooth brushing) and bleeding complications in previous surgery can be revealed if the patient is awake. Information about current medication with aspirin or clopidogrel is important, along with the most recent INR and ACT values and platelet count.

12.4.2.2 Physical Examination

Early postoperative bleeding is noted as a subcutaneous hematoma under the skin incision. Often it rapidly increases in size. Marking the limits of the hematoma with a permanent marker pen is a good way to facilitate estimating such expansion. Bleeding from incisions is another common presentation and is often revealed when nurses need to change dressings frequently or when more than 50 ml/h of blood is emptied from a drain. Bleeding occurring after the first postoperative days is usually associated with signs of infection at physical examination. The patient can often inform the physician about infection and bleeding problems in the surgical wound (Table 12.3).

Postoperative bleeding in the abdomen after major surgical procedures, such as aortic surgery, is difficult to diagnose. Medical history, signs of hypovolemia, and laboratory tests are helpful but imprecise (Table 12.3). Dilated intestines, which normally are seen after aortic surgery, make examination of the abdomen difficult. In obese patients it is almost impossible to interpret findings. Intestinal bleeding after aortic surgery is a sign of a intestinal ischemia and has already been discussed above.

Table 12.3. Factors suggesting hemorrhage that requires reoperation after aortic surgery

Tachycardia (>100/min for 15 min)
Hypotension (<90 mmHg for 15 min)
Increasing abdominal circumference
Acute or complicated primary operation
Hemoglobin concentration not rising despite transfusion of red blood cells

12.4.3 Diagnostics

Postoperative bleeding does not require diagnostic work-up. The only exception is intestinal bleeding after aortic surgery; this situation has already been discussed.

12.4.4 Management and Treatment

12.4.4.1 In the Emergency Department, ICU, or Surgical Ward

Emergency Measures

Profuse bleeding from a wound can be temporarily controlled by finger compression while the patient is being transported to the operating room. Additionally, in large hemorrhages causing hypovolemia, packed cells and fresh-frozen plasma are given to the patient. Fresh-frozen plasma contains coagulation factors that are consumed during bleeding, and it decreases the risk for a disturbed hemostasis. If overly generous preoperative or intraoperative administration of heparin is suspected to be a contributing factor to the bleeding, its effect could be reversed by protamine. Such treatment should be avoided if possible, and heparin's effects are probably overestimated as a cause for bleedings; the effect of heparin in plasma is decreased by 50% within 90 min. Three hours postoperatively, only 25% remains to affect the coagulation system. Too rapid infusion of protamine can induce hypotension because of diminished cardiac function. Furthermore, a slight overdose might cause thrombosis of small-caliber grafts. If bleeding persists and there are no good alternative treatment options, 10 mg of protamine dissolved in 15 ml of saline can be administered over 10 min.

Which Patients Should be Reoperated?

A basic principle is that patients who are bleeding and display some signs of hypovolemia, such as tachycardia and a blood pressure less than 100 mmHg for a while, shall be re-operated emergently. This is also true for hematomas that doubled its size within 30 minutes as well as drain bleedings exceeding 50–70 ml/h. These guidelines, however, are not generally valid and each patient has to be individually evaluated.

The rationale for reoperation and evacuation of hematomas is the risk for graft compression and postoperative infection. Other indications for evacuating a hematoma are severe pain due to compression of nerves and extensively distended skin with risk for perforation. Evacuation operations should always be performed under sterile conditions in an operating room. This is particularly important for bleeding with a coexisting infection. A new dose of antibiotic prophylaxis should be given to all patients needing reoperation for bleeding.

Bleeding After Aortic Surgery

Patients with signs of hypovolemia after aortic operations should be reoperated with wide indications (Table 12.3). Such reoperations might become difficult and experienced assistance is often valuable. Besides being difficult to diagnose, the bleeding site is also often hard to identify, get access to, and repair during the reoperation.

Substantial hemorrhage during the primary operation can cause a deficiency in coagulation factors. Before starting the reoperation, it is recommended to check if the patient has received packed cells. If the amount administered exceeded four to six units, at least two units of fresh frozen plasma should be given right away. If more than eight units of red blood cells had been given, a thrombocytopenia may contribute to the bleeding.

Bleeding During Thrombolysis

The treatment of bleeding from a puncture site after angiography or thrombolysis follows the principles outlined above. After thrombolysis is completed, the introducer is usually left in place until the thrombolytic agent's activity has diminished.

An oozing bleeding around the introducer during thrombolysis requires special attention. In most cases local compression around the catheter is sufficient to stop the bleeding and to allow continued thrombolysis. A prerequisite is that the fibrinogen concentration systemically is >1 g/l. If fibrinogen levels are lower, and also if bleeding occurs in other locations, infusion of the thrombolytic agent should be stopped.

Medical Treatment and Observation Only

Minor bleeding from surgical wounds and small hematomas is observed with applied compression over the area. For prolonged minor bleeding, hemoglobin, INR and ACT values, and platelet count are checked, and medications affecting the coagulation system are discontinued. These blood samples have a low sensitivity as a screening test for hemostasic function and only 30% of normal co-agulation activity is required to obtain normal values. A better measure of platelet function is the number of platelets or the bleeding time. A prolonged bleeding time supports the use of desmopressin. If a disturbed hemostasis without obvious causes is found, consultation with a coagulation specialist is recommended. A platelet count $<50 \times 10^9$/l is considered insufficient for hemostasis and is an indication for platelet transfusion in case of bleeding. At reoperations platelets should be administered immediately before the start of the operation to give the best possible effect.

12.4.4.2 Operation

Control of Bleeding

Profuse bleeding sometimes needs compression over the bleeding site while the patient is being scrubbed and draped for surgery. Compression must be applied proximal to the bleeding site to allow scrubbing if it is in the groin. For more distal incisional bleedings, a tourniquet achieves control. After opening the skin, an assistant compresses the inflow artery with a "peanut" or "strawberry" and keeps the wound free from blood with suction to facilitate exposure. In bleeding episodes after endovascular procedures, proximal control is best obtained cranial to the puncture site, which mostly is in the groin, to avoid dissection through blood-embedded tissue. The technique has been described in Chapters 9 (p. 107) and 15 (p. 180).

Bleeding from or in the vicinity of the proximal anastomosis of aortic surgery is sometimes challenging. In general, clamping the aorta is necessary to obtain control. If the reason for the bleeding is a soft and weak posterior wall of the aorta there is a substantial risk that even a slight pull on the graft will disrupt the suture line. If there is major bleeding from this region temporary subdiaphragmatic aortic control should be obtained before attempting to repair the suture row (see also Chapter 7). Other possible sites for arterial bleeding after AAA surgery are the anastomosis of the lumbar arteries in the aneurysmal sac and the inferior mesenteric artery. Anastomoses are also possible bleeding sites. Venous bleeding after aortic aneurysm surgery comes from the iliac veins or lumbar veins at the level of the proximal anastomosis.

Repair of Bleeding Sites

Anastomotic bleedings and minor puncture bleedings in grafts or arteries are best controlled by simple sutures. It is important to avoid applying bites and stitches that are too large because that may cause tears and reduce the vessel lumen. Placing the sutures and tying them with the artery clamped decrease the risk for tears. Bleeding from a vein graft branch caused by a slipped ligature should be repaired with prolene suturing rather than another attempt with ligation. Vascular clamps that are too strong may cause perforation of the graft wall. It is better to use rubber-reinforced clamps or vessel loops.

When major hemorrhage is under control the entire operating field is searched for minor bleedings. Every single bleeding site should be controlled by electrocautery. Hematomas are also evacuated. Continued bleeding from the wound edges suggests a disturbed coagulation system; if it occurs, coagulation tests and platelet counts are rechecked. Administration of more fresh frozen plasma might be indicated.

In some circumstances hemostasis can be facilitated by local measures. Examples are cellulose sheets (Surgicel^{tm}), which after contact with blood swells and produces a gelatinous substance and that mechanically facilitates coagulation. Another alternative is sheets of collagen (Avitene^{tm} and Lyostypt^{tm}), which enhance local adhesion of platelets. Another effective but rather expensive possibility is to use fibrin glue (Tissel^{tm}) or preparations of thrombin (FlowSeal^{tm}) to cover the raw surface and thereby seal bleeding minor vessels.

Bleeding associated with infection should be treated by ligature of the graft. Synthetic grafts should be removed entirely, with vein patching to cover remaining defects in the artery.

12.4.4.3 Management After Treatment

Patients who have undergone reoperations for bleeding should, of course, be monitored postoperatively for continued bleeding. This is of great importance if the cause it has not been identified. Hemoglobin concentration and platelet counts are checked every 4th hour, and after major bleeding replacement with packed cells and fresh frozen plasma is continued. Patients requiring reoperation because of bleeding after aortic surgery are at risk of developing multiple organ failure and are treated in the ICU. They also suffer an increased risk of developing ischemic colitis.

12.5 Infections

12.5.1 Pathophysiology

12.5.1.1 Types of Infection

The most common postoperative infection complicating vascular surgery is wound infection. It is benign, local, has few systemic effects, and responds well to local treatment and antibiotics. The most common localization is in groin incisions, followed by thigh and calf. If left untreated, wound infections can spread and engage subcutaneous tissue. Eventually the graft may be involved, which is a serious complication. Graft infections might occur any time postoperatively and have been reported as late as 15 years after the primary procedure. A combination of surgical and antibiotic treatment is sometimes successful. The surgical treatment includes total extirpation of the graft, and in many cases the distal perfusion has to be restored by extraanatomical reconstructions routed away from the infected area. The most feared and challenging infectious complication occurs when an aortic graft is engaged. Aortic graft infection is a major diagnostic problem, and the 30 day mortality is as high as 50%.

Table 12.4. Risk factors for development of vascular graft infection

General	Systemic
Emergency operation	Diabetes
Reoperation	Cortisone treatment
Inadequate sterile technique	Malignancy
Long operating time	Leukopenia
Simultaneous gastro-intestinal operation	Malnutrition
Postoperative wound infection	Chemotherapy
Remote infection	Chronic renal insufficiency

12.5.1.2 Microbiology

The vascular graft and the surgical wound become contaminated with bacteria systemically or by direct contact during the operation. Hematoma and leakage of lymph and other wound secretions, especially in diabetic patients, are all perfect media for bacterial growth. The virulence of the bacteria and the patient's general condition determine the course of the infection and its severity. There is also a possible correlation between bacterial virulence and the time when the infection occurs. Early infections, within 30 days of the primary surgery, tend to be more serious and are often caused by more virulent organisms such as Staphylococcus aureus and Gram-negative bacteria. Late infections are caused by coagulase-negative staphylococci of low virulence. There is an ongoing debate about the significance of these bacteria. Some argue that they rarely are responsible for graft infections, that this a common contamination of the wound, and that the unspecific symptoms and findings typical for these "low-virulence" infections instead represent an inflammatory reaction to the graft material. This concept is supported by the fact that less aggressive treatment usually is more effective in coagulase-negative staphylococci infections compared with those caused by a more virulent bacteria. Wound infections are mostly caused by Staphylococcus aureus.

12.5.1.3 Pathophysiology

Besides constituting a risk for septicemia and a threat to graft function, infections also imply a risk for bleeding by erosion of arterial and graft walls, including the anastomosis. Such erosions can, even if they are small, lead to life-threatening hemorrhage and to the development of pseudo-aneurysms. If such bleeding occurs in the proximal anastomosis of an aortic reconstruction it will most likely be profuse and lethal. A special type of erosion-related bleeding is seen when an aortoduodenal fistula develops. It results from an erosion that creates a communication between the aorta and the duodenum. It presents as gastrointestinal bleeding, and blood cultures are often positive for intestinal bacteria. The bleeding usually starts as a minor, deceptively innocent hematemesis or rectal bleeding, followed by several days without symptoms. This "herald bleeding" is probably secondary to the erosion of the duodenal wall. When the

fistula is established, sooner or later a massive and often lethal hemorrhage occurs. An alternative explanation for the pathophysiology of aortoduodenal fistula infections is mechanical tear. The main argument for this is that the aortic pulsations cause movements between the anastomosis and the duodenum that erode the intestinal wall until it perforates and contaminates the graft.

12.5.2 Clinical Presentation

Wound infections are easy to recognize. Accordingly, it is aortic graft infections that will be the main subject of the following paragraphs. A high level of suspicion is needed to even consider aortic graft infection because the clinical presentation is diffuse and general. It should be suspected in patients who have atypical symptoms. The diagnosis is most difficult in a low-virulent graft infection.

12.5.2.1 Medical History

Besides information about the primary operation, the patient should be asked about unspecific general symptoms such as fatigue, loss of appetite, weight loss, nausea, and low-grade fever. The circumstances around the primary operation are important, and operations that were long in duration, complicated, and done as an emergency, support the suspicion of graft infection. A superficial wound infection immediately after the primary operation should also alert the examiner. Symptoms of gastrointestinal bleeding are an alarming sign in patients who have undergone aortic reconstructions and the diagnosis of aortoduodenal fistula should always be suspected until disproved.

The patient should also be asked about tenderness, delayed healing of surgical wounds, and the presence of swelling or masses in the operation area. The latter can be the sign of a pseudoaneurysm or abscess. It is also important to ask about secretions from the scars.

12.5.2.2 Physical Examination

In addition to a general physical examination, including graft function, the operation wound is examined with special emphasis on infection signs and secretions (Fig. 12.2). Also, the areas around the scars need to be investigated for fistulas, pulsating masses, and tender swellings. If an infected

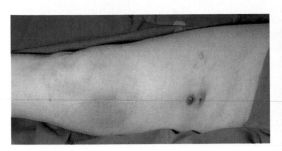

Fig. 12.2. Clinical signs of graft infection following infrainguinal bypass surgery

surgical wound is open due to dehiscence or debridement it is important to examine whether the graft is visible. A visible graft often necessitates graft removal.

12.5.2.3 Laboratory Tests

In wound infections and local infections engaging smaller grafts, laboratory tests are not needed to establish the diagnosis.

In aortic graft infections laboratory tests usually suggest a pronounced systemic infection with leukocyte counts $>15 \times 10^9/l$ and high C-reactive protein values. The amount of increase, however, varies with the grade of infection. When presentation is vague, additional laboratory tests such as differential count or electrophoresis can occasionally facilitate differentiation from other diseases. Test results can be normal during infections caused by coagulase-negative staphylococci. Patients often also have a slight anemia and low albumin levels in serum. Stools should be checked for the presence of blood when aortic graft infections are suspected. The value of this can, however, be debated because the specificity in diagnoses of occult bleeding from aortoduodenal fistulas is low.

12.5.3 Diagnostics

Ultrasound can reveal the presence of fluid collections close to the graft or anastomosis and differentiate hematomas from aneurysms. A special problem is deciding how much fluid can be considered normal around grafts recently implanted. The fluid should be absorbed within 3–6 weeks, but before that time, fluid collections can be considered normal findings.

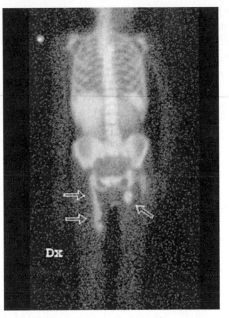

Fig. 12.3. An example of a positive leukocyte scintigram. *Arrows* point toward areas with suspected infection

12.5.3.1 Aortic Graft Infection

The first investigation done to reveal signs of aortic graft infection is CT. The question to be answered is whether there is fluid or gas around the graft and inside the aneurysm sac. The normal postoperative course is that fluid and gas should be absorbed within 3–6 weeks. Accordingly, gas bubbles around the graft after 20 days postoperatively suggest that infection is a possible diagnosis. Unfortunately, it is not always easy to differentiate from intestinal gas. Magnetic resonance imaging (MRI) is an alternative for the work-up. It is better for differentiating between fluid collections, old thrombi, and inflammatory changes in tissue. Unless the diagnosis is obvious after the initial investigation, most patients with suspected aortic graft infections are examined with both CT and MRI. Our recommendation is that CT is ordered first when aortoduodenal fistula is suspected, and MRI is ordered for all other patients. Other methods such as a leukocyte scintigram can be helpful when CT and MRI are unable to establish the diagnosis (Fig. 12.3).

Table 12.5. Diagnostic methods used for aortic graft infections

Method	Sensitivity	Specificity	Comment
Computed tomography	57–94%	85–100%	Best results in aortoduodenal fistula
Magnetic resonance imaging	85%	100%	For primary graft infections
Leukocyte scintigram	80–100%	50–85%	For primary graft infections and aortoduodenal fistulas

Patients with a history of gastrointestinal bleeding should be examined with endoscopy. It is important to view the entire duodenum all the way down to the distal part, which usually is located close to the anastomotic area in the aorta and where blood clots or ongoing bleeding are most likely to be found. An examination that fails to include this part of the duodenum is incomplete. Occasionally, graft material can be seen through a defect in the mucosa. A normal examination, on the other hand, does not exclude aortoduodenal fistula. Unfortunately, none of the diagnostic methods mentioned above can exclude the diagnosis of graft infection (Table 12.4).

When the patient presents with mild symptoms a lot of time is available for further diagnostic work-up, such as technetium or leukocyte scintigrams (Table 12.5). When the patient has groin sinus and fistula, a fistulogram can be done by injecting contrast. This can map the sinus system and disclose whether it connects with the graft. Angiography does not add any information for establishing the diagnosis but is sometimes needed for planning the reconstruction after removal of an infected graft.

12.5.4 Management and Treatment

12.5.4.1 In the Emergency Department

Wound and subcutaneous graft infections

Patients with wound infections should be admitted to the ward for observation because of the risk for graft involvement and bleeding. Only very mild and superficial infections can be treated in the outpatient clinic. Wound debridement should never be performed in the outpatient clinic or emergency department. Antibiotic treatment is started after samples for microbiological cultures are obtained. Because Staphylococcus aureus is the most common bacteria, oral cloxacillin is given. If the patient has diabetes or if the wound is suspected to be contaminated with intestinal bacteria, antibiotics with a broader efficacy spectrum are recommended.

For deeper infections, especially if a graft is involved, the patient needs surgery as soon as possible. If the patient is septic and has impaired circulation, immediate surgery is indicated irrespective of the time of day. The first dose of antibiotics should be administered intravenously in the emergency department. When deciding if it is enough to drain an abscess or if graft extirpation is necessary, a duplex examination can reveal whether an infected hematoma is connected to the graft. Graft extirpation is usually indicated when a synthetic graft is visible in a ruptured surgical wound. An exposed vein graft must be ligated to prevent bleeding. In cases with deeper infections involving autologous or synthetic grafts the patient is admitted to the ward and treated with antibiotics even if he or she has mild symptoms. If a patient with a synthetic graft infection still has fever and signs of remaining infection in laboratory tests after 2–3 days of treatment, extirpation of the graft is also indicated. This is valid even with diminished signs of local infection.

Suspected Aortoduodenal Fistula

Patients with a previous aortic procedure, a recent history of gastrointestinal bleeding, and an impaired general condition should be suspected to have an aortic graft infection. Accordingly, they are candidates for observation and treatment in the ICU. There is a risk for massive acute bleeding and careful monitoring of cardiac and renal function is necessary. For such patients it is essential to have IV lines inserted and packed red cells available for transfusion if bleeding occurs. Blood cultures and other cultures should be obtained before antibiotic therapy is started. If the patient's condition allows, investigations with endoscopy, duplex or CT scanning are performed. If such a patient has ongoing significant bleeding and shows signs of prolonged hypovolemia, he or she must immediately be transported to the operating room. It is also important to call for assistance. Aortic graft infection hemorrhage is one of the major challenges in vascular surgery and vast experience is necessary to have some chance to save the patient. Fortunately this complication is very rare, occurring after only 0.1–0.2% of all aortic reconstructions.

Other Aortic Graft Infections

Patients with suspected graft infection in the abdomen and mild symptoms are admitted to the ward for daytime work-up. If the suspicion is strong, such as in cases with purulent secretion from the groin, antibiotic therapy should be started immediately. Investigations include CT or MRI to verify the diagnosis to reveal if the graft is engaged and to plan an upcoming surgical procedure. The surgical strategy often includes complicated procedures even in cases of less dramatic infections. The most common is an axillobifemoral bypass to ensure circulation to the lower extremities, followed by a second procedure during which the entire aortic graft is removed.

12.5.4.2 Operation

Control

In graft infections in the extremities, proximal and distal control is obtained by separate incisions through unaffected tissue. Synthetic grafts, for instance, must be controlled by exposure and banding of inflow as well as outflow vessels, including all branches. This is easy when the graft is surrounded by pus but difficult if the dissection must be performed through scar tissue.

Control of the aorta during graft infection surgery is very difficult. Because of the risk for massive bleeding it should not be attempted – unless absolutely necessary – if experience is limited. It involves a long mid line incision and clamping of the aorta subdiaphragmatically, either manually or with a straight clamp applied through the mi-

nor omentum (Chapter 7, p. 83). Control can also be achieved by balloon insertion from the groin or brachial artery (page 83). Once proximal control has been achieved resuscitation is continued while waiting for the arrival of experienced assistance.

Continued Operation

Irrespective of strategy the continued operation usually requires experience in vascular surgery with the possible exception of vein graft ligation. Easiest is to divide the graft between two vascular clamps proximal to the infected area and suture-ligate both ends with prolene sutures. Such ligatures should preferably be placed in fresh, not infected, tissue. Synthetic grafts should be totally extirpated and the defects in the native arteries covered with patches of autologous vein. It is usually necessary to restore the circulation in the extremity. In graft infections in the lower extremities it is common to try to delay immediate reconstruction and wait until the infection has healed, but this often increases the risk for amputation.

The continued operation in aortic graft infections is complicated and requires vascular surgical expertise. Several alternatives are possible and the type of infection, its extension, and the availability of new graft material from the patient determines the choice. In many cases the old graft has to be totally extirpated; the aortic, iliac, and femoral stumps oversewn; and the circulation of the lower extremity restored extraanatomically, usually by an axillobifemoral bypass. Other cases can be reconstructed in situ with vein grafts, thrombectomized arteries, or homologous or synthetic grafts. In infections of seemingly low virulence, only partial excision of grafts can be considered. Local antibiotic treatment is then common as part of the management.

Samples for aerobic as well as anaerobic microbiological cultures should be obtained from the operation field as well as from excised grafts. The wound should never be left open for secondary healing with an exposed vascular graft. All segments of patent grafts must be covered with soft tissue.

12.5.4.3 Management After Treatment

Antibiotic treatment should be continued postoperatively even if the infected graft has been removed. Open wounds need daily control and dressing changes to avoid spreading or persisting infection. Patients operated for aortic graft infection are treated in the ICU postoperatively. They require careful monitoring of all vital organs, including perfusion of the extremities.

12.5.5 Results and Outcome

Reported results of treatment of graft infections clearly demonstrate that such infections are dangerous and complicated to treat. Thirty-day mortality after surgery for graft infections in the extremities is reported to be in the range of 10–17%, with an amputation rate of 40%. The variability of the results depends on the choice of treatment method. If only a ligature of an infected graft is done, the risk of a new infection and postoperative bleedings is low, approximately 5%. But at least 25% of patients have amputations within 30 days. If, on the other hand, graft excision and a new vascular reconstruction are performed in situ after local treatment with antibiotics, a new infection and serious bleeding will occur in about 30% of patients. The amputation risk is only 6% and is substantially less than with graft ligation.

Early mortality in primary aortic graft infections is 25% after the surgical treatment, and 20% of patients will lose at least one leg. The mortality for patients with aortoduodenal fistulas is almost 50%. Extraanatomical bypass construction before graft excision appears to improve the results considerably compared with simultaneous extirpation and reconstruction.

12.6 Local Complications

12.6.1 Lymphocele and Seroma

12.6.1.1 Background and Causes
Subcutaneous fluid collections in wounds are common postoperatively, especially in the groin. When a collection is discovered within 24 h after the procedure it is usually a hematoma, but when a well-demarcated fluid collection appears later during the first postoperative weeks, it is a seroma or lymphocele. Such swellings are created when degraded blood products and tissue secretions accumulate in the wound – a seroma – or when

lymph vessels or glands are damaged during dissection and the lymph collections are built up – a lymphocele. Both types have the potential to spontaneously be absorbed or drained through the incision. In the latter case a lymph fistula is created and drainage of lymph will go on intermittently for several weeks. Lymphocele is reported to occur in 1–6% of all groin incisions. Both of these complications can transform into manifest infection and are therefore associated with an increased risk for postoperative wound and graft infection.

12.6.1.2 Clinical Presentation
Seroma and lymphocele can be difficult to differentiate from early wound infection. A fluctuating mass that is easy to delineate by palpation is a typical finding. The area around the incision is swollen but not tender and red. A clear fluid might ooze from the incision. The amount of drained fluid is generally considerable and the patient often states that the dressing has to be changed several times a day to keep the area dry and clean. Ultrasound is sometimes required to differentiate hematoma from lymphocele.

12.6.1.3 Management and Treatment
Surveillance is the best management for most cases of fluid collections. A majority are absorbed spontaneously and also when fistulation occurs. Much patience is needed in cases with lymph leakage because the healing process may take several months.

Because seromas and lymphoceles are likely to increase the risk for infection the literature advocates active exploration and evacuation of all large postoperative fluid collections. A selective approach is more common, however. This management strategy suggests surgical treatment only for wounds with heavy secretion and those suspected to be related to synthetic grafts. The operation includes evacuating the fluid and covering the graft with tissue, frequently by applying several rows of absorbable sutures. Old long-lasting lymphoceles have a capsule that should be excised after ligation of afferent lymph vessels.

12.6.2 Postoperative Leg Swelling

12.6.2.1 Background and Causes

After successful vascular reconstruction for lower extremity ischemia over half of all patients will suffer from more or less pronounced swelling of the operated leg. Indeed, many vascular surgeons argue that this is a reliable sign of a successful operation. Patients with severe ischemia are the ones who will swell the most. The explanation for this complication is not clear, but a disturbed microcirculation, a diffuse venous thrombosis, impaired lymph drainage, and reperfusion have all been suggested as possible causes. The swelling usually increases successively and reaches its maximum 2–3 weeks after reconstruction and can be expected to last several months.

12.6.2.2 Clinical Presentation

Because the leg is heavy, numb, stiff, and aching, the patient is usually worried about it. The edema is localized to the calf and foot and is apparent at physical examination on the 2nd or 3rd postoperative day. This usually coincides in time with the patient's resumption of ambulation. The swelling is most pronounced at the ankle level, but the entire leg can be involved. The diagnosis is easy to establish, but in some cases a duplex scan is required to differentiate this condition from deep venous thrombosis. Duplex scanning is recommended for the patient who, in addition to the swelling, develops cyanosis or tenderness over the calf muscles or has a severe and inexplicable pain in the leg.

12.6.2.3 Management and Treatment

The leg swelling needs no specific treatment other than elevation and patience. This treatment is also sufficient when the swelling persists longer than 2 months after the operation. Other contributing causes, such as cardiac failure, should, of course, be corrected if possible. Compression stockings with mild compression could also be tried to relieve the symptoms. Mannitol, furosemide, and allopurinol have all been tried with no documented effect. An important aspect is to inform the patient about the benign nature of this condition.

12.6.3 Wound Edge Necrosis

12.6.3.1 Background and Causes

Wound edge necrosis is a complication that affects calf incisions used for distal reconstructions. It is caused by ischemia in the wound edges. Some studies indicates that up to 15% of all procedures will be troubled by wound edge necrosis. Risk factors are a long operating time, severe ischemia, and the application of self-retaining retractors that are too strong. Surgical undermining of the skin and subcutaneous tissue during the operation also increases the risk.

12.6.3.2 Clinical Presentation

A few days postoperatively a red or bluish discoloration of the skin along the wound edges is noted. The discoloration can be partial, but the extent usually increases during the following day and might occasionally engage the entire incision. The discolored area is slowly transformed into black necrosis without displaying signs of infection. Within a week the necrosis is clearly demarcated against normally perfused and vital skin. This condition is often combined with a successful reconstruction and a swollen leg. It is important to differentiate this dry necrosis from the more serious ischemic necrosis with wound breakdown, dehiscence, and overt infection that was discussed previously in this chapter.

12.6.3.3 Management and Treatment

Wound necrosis usually heals by itself through ingrowth of new skin from the wound edges. With time it will cover the entire wound surface. A prerequisite for healing is that the necrosis be loosened and surgically removed. The healing process might occasionally require several months and, in rare cases, a split skin graft when the necrosis is large. Accordingly, active treatment consists of superficial wound revision and dressing changes.

12.6.4 Local Nerve Injuries

12.6.4.1 Background and Causes

Sensory and motor nerve injuries are common after carotid surgery and occur distal to groin and calf incisions after vascular reconstruction in the leg. The lumbosacral plexus and the main stem of the femoral nerve can also be injured during aortic and iliac vascular surgery. Stripping of the greater saphenous vein below the knee is also associated with a high risk for injuries to the saphenous nerve, which is why distal stripping is avoided nowadays. The mechanism of injury during all of these procedures is usually division or ischemic damage secondary to pressure from retractors during the procedure. Occasionally a hematoma can compress and affect the nerve.

12.6.4.2 Clinical Presentation

The patient usually describes a numb and painful skin area within the dermatome of the injured nerve. The pain in nerve injuries is burning and often combined with hyperesthesia. Some examples of injured nerves and the corresponding skin area affected are listed in Table 12.6.

Table 12.6. Injured nerves and corresponding symptomatic skin areas

Damaged nerve	Symptomatic area
Major auricular nerve	Skin around the ear lobe
Branches to the femoral nerve	Medial skin of the thigh
Saphenous nerve	Skin medially below the knee and of the foot
Lumbosacral plexus	Unilateral or bilateral motor and sensory deficits in large areas of the legs

12.6.4.3 Management and Treatment

There is no effective treatment for these types of nerve injuries. The patient should be informed that the injury is benign despite its nuisance, and that it might heal and disappear with time. Peripheral nerves have a considerable capacity for regeneration and the symptoms can be expected to successively decrease up to at least 1 year after the operation. The same is valid for mainstem injuries. Patients in whom the pain is considerable should be offered analgesics and possibly also a nerve block.

■ Further Reading

Adam DJ, Haggart PC, Ludlam CA, et al. Coagulopathy and hyperfibrinolysis in ruptured abdominal aortic aneurysm repair. Ann Vasc Surg 2004; 18(5):572–577

Cherry KJ Jr, Roland CF, Pairolero PC, et al. Infected femorodistal bypass: is graft removal mandatory? J Vasc Surg 1992; 15(2):295–303

Drews RE. Critical issues in hematology: anemia, thrombocytopenia, coagulopathy, and blood product transfusions in critically ill patients. Clin Chest Med 2003; 24(4):607–622

de Figueiredo LF, Coselli JS. Individual strategies of hemostasis for thoracic aortic surgery. J Card Surg 1997; 12(2 Suppl):222–228

Fujitani RM. Revision of the failing vein graft: outcome of secondary operations. Semin Vasc Surg 1993; 6(2):118–129

Kuestner LM, Reilly LM, Jicha DL, et al. Secondary aortoenteric fistula: contemporary outcome with use of extraanatomic bypass and infected graft excision. J Vasc Surg 1995; 21(2):184–195

Schwartz ML, Veith FJ, Panetta TF, et al. Reoperative approaches for failed infrainguinal polytetrafluoroethylene (PTFE) grafts. Semin Vasc Surg 1994; 7(3):165–172

Taylor SM, Weatherford DA, Langan EM, et al. Outcomes in the management of vascular prosthetic graft infections confined to the groin: a reappraisal. Ann Vasc Surg 1996; 10(2):117–122

Young RM, Cherry KJ Jr, Davis PM, et al. The results of in situ prosthetic replacement for infected aortic grafts. Am J Surg 1999; 178(2):136–140

Acute Venous Problems

13

CONTENTS

13.1 Summary

- Thrombolysis is a viable treatment option for patients with deep vein thrombosis.
- Phlegmasia cerulea dolens may require surgical thrombectomy or thrombolysis as well as fasciotomy
- Use of a cava filter when indicated may save patients from pulmonary embolism
- Patients with thrombophlebitis extending into the deep venous system may require surgical ligation of the greater saphenous vein.

13.2 Background and Pathogenesis

13.2.1 Background

The main scope of this chapter is to discuss miscellaneous venous problems, mainly thromboembolic disease, but not venous injuries. The latter is covered in Part 1 of this book which focuses on specific regions of the body.

As listed in the incidence table below (Table 13.1), venous thrombosis is quite common. The

Table 13.1. Incidence of venous thromboembolism (*PE* pulmonary embolism, *DVT* deep vein thrombosis)

Country	Year assessed	Type of disease	Population age (years)	Incidence per 100,000 persons per year
USA (California)	1996	30% PE 70% DVT	Adults 15–80	90
Sweden	1991–2000	59% PE 41% DVT	Women 15–44	36
USA (Minnesota)	1966–1990	59% PE 41% DVT	Adults (hospital based)	117
Italy	Before 2000	19% PE 80% DVT (lower limb) 1% DVT (upper limb)	Adults 18–65	77

incidence varies with the population studied and increases with age. Hospital-based studies present a larger proportion of pulmonary embolism (PE), whereas community cohorts have more thrombosis patients. Manifestations range from a superficial thrombophlebitis or a minor deep venous thrombosis (DVT) that produces only minute symptoms to a DVT with massive embolism to the lungs, threatening the patient's life. While open surgical treatment of venous thromboembolic disease is rarely indicated, it is helpful to have basic knowledge about diagnosis, pathogenesis, and anticoagulation treatment. This is important for differential diagnosis and for the few instances when emergency endovascular or open surgical treatment is indicated. This chapter will also describe the technique for surgical and endovascular treatment of acute DVT.

13.2.2 Pathogenesis

When DVT occurs, clots have usually formed in the small deep veins in the calf. Patients afflicted have hypercoagulative disorders, are taking medications that affect clotting that make them susceptible to venous thrombosis, has malignancy or has been immobilized for a larger period. The clot causes a local inflammation in the venous wall and adjacent tissue that may make the calf tender. Because the small veins in the calf are paired, the clot does not cause significant venous obstruction or distal edema. Flow in the obstructed vein will decrease, however, which increases the risk for continuing clot formation. The clot will then grow in a proximal direction and continue to obstruct more veins. Also at this stage distal edema is quite uncommon because collateral flow is extensive in the legs, and significant swelling does not occur until the common femoral vein is obstructed. At this level the outflow from the deep femoral, superficial, and great saphenous vein is affected. Continued obstruction, causing near occlusion of all the main veins in the leg and pelvis, can lead to a dreaded condition called phlegmasia cerulea dolens (discussed later). Any time during this process there is also a substantial risk that clots will dislodge from the leg veins, follow the blood flow to the lungs, and cause PE.

Primary iliac vein thrombosis occurs most commonly on the left side where a stenosis frequently is a predisposing factor.

13.3 Clinical Presentation

Patients with DVT experience pain and leg swelling that often is worse when standing or walking. Some patients also feel warmth and notice that the leg is red. Patients with caval obstruction have bilateral symptoms. These examples constitute the classic symptoms of DVT, but many patients do not have any symptoms at all and present with PE only. Signs of this condition include shortness of breath and chest pain that may be worsened by deep breaths. Occasionally, patients also report that they have been coughing up phlegm that may be tinged with blood.

Patients with phlegmasia cerulea dolens have similar but more severe symptoms. Discoloration is often pronounced. Pedal pulses are usually absent, and the leg is very tender. Foot gangrene is also noted occasionally. It may therefore be mistaken for arterial embolism, but misdiagnosis can be avoided by remembering that acute arterial occlusion does not cause edema.

Physical examination is only 30% accurate for DVT and a poor way to establish the diagnosis. The most common finding, however, is localized calf tenderness. Homan's sign – pain when dorsiflexing the foot with the knee extended – is neither sensitive nor specific and should probably not be used. Other examination findings are visible superficial collateral veins, pitting edema, and swelling of the entire leg. To be significant, the latter should expand the calf circumference by more than 3 cm compared with the other leg.

Patients with primary iliac vein thrombosis may present with abdominal pain in the lower quadrant, tenderness over the vascular bundle in the groin and general swelling of the leg.

Patients with upper limb thrombosis have similar symptoms; the most common are arm swelling and discoloration or pain.

Scoring systems combining clinical findings and medical history have been proposed to increase accuracy of the examination. If the examination is positive for more than three of the signs and symptoms described above, up to 75% of the patients have evidence of DVT as diagnosed by duplex examination.

13.4 Diagnostics

All patients, including those considered to have only small risk to be suffering from DVT and those having arm symptoms, should undergo duplex scanning or perhaps phlebography. The duplex examination includes visualization of the veins, clots, blood flow, and vein compressibility. The latter is considered a direct test of DVT because a vein with clot cannot be compressed, whereas the walls of a healthy vein are very easy to squeeze together by pressure with the probe. Lack of blood flow variation with breathing is another sign suggesting DVT on duplex examination. Phlebography includes cannulating a superficial foot vein and injecting contrast during fluoroscopy to enable visualization of thrombosed veins. This method was the standard diagnostic procedure before duplex appeared as the primary choice for establishing the DVT diagnosis. Today it is used mostly when duplex is unavailable in the hospital or when it is unable to identify the deep leg veins.

Another test useful for DVT diagnosis is determining the concentration of the fibrin degradation product D-dimer in the blood. This test has a sensitivity for DVT of 90% or greater as well as a negative predictive value of 90% or greater by most studies. Accordingly, a negative D-dimer level (the cut-off level depends on the type of assay used) in a symptomatic patient with a clinically suspected diagnosis nearly provides exclusion of DVT. Therefore, it is suitable as a screening test before further work-up when the diagnosis is not obvious.

13.5 Management and Treatment

13.5.1 In the Emergency Department

Patients who complain of unilateral limb swelling and pain should be suspected to have DVT and have a blood sample drawn for measuring D-dimer. A negative test excludes DVT or PE as the primary diagnosis. Patients with a positive D-dimer may suffer from a venous thromboembolic disease and need further work-up. In most hospi-

tals this means starting with duplex scanning to establish the diagnosis. If signs of DVT are present, it is important to elucidate the extent of thrombosis during the examination. This information is useful in the management process because some patients with femoral vein, iliac vein, or cava thrombosis may need thrombolysis or even a cava filter. When the DVT diagnosis is confirmed, baseline blood coagulation parameters are obtained, and low molecular weight heparin treatment is initiated. It is also important to exclude other diagnoses that could contribute to the thrombosis formation. For example, clinical indications of an intraabdominal malignancy could be confirmed or eliminated by computed tomography (CT). Both inpatient and outpatient protocols can then be used for the continued treatment of the patients. (No further recommendations will be given on the medical management of DVT here because this book is intended to focus on vascular surgical treatment.)

Few diagnosed patients are candidates for urgent surgical or endovascular treatment, but the most common situations when it can be considered are listed in Table 13.2. Patients with upper limb thrombosis may also benefit from urgent thrombolysis. The same clinical findings listed in the table are also applicable in patients with duplex-verified axillary or subclavian vein thrombosis.

If D-dimer is positive and pulmonary symptoms are prominent in the medical history (or the

Table 13.2. Clinical findings indicating that open surgical or endovascular treatment should be considered in patients with duplex-verified thrombosis into femoral and/or iliac veins

Clinical findings	Treatment type(s)
Young age	Thrombolysis
Duration of symptoms <10 days	Thrombolysis
Pronounced symptoms	Thrombolysis
Contraindications to heparin treatment	Cava filter, thrombectomy
Phlegmasia cerulea dolens	Thrombolysis, thrombectomy, fasciotomy
Free-floating thrombus in vena cava	Cava filter

patient has chest pain or hemoptysis), a CT scan is added to the duplex and laboratory work-up to reveal signs of PE. Furthermore, if PE is confirmed, evaluation of the heart function by echocardiography is also valuable. Such patients should also receive oxygen. It must be kept in mind that patients with PE may have a negative D-dimer. If suspicion is strong, the work-up should proceed regardless of the outcome of this test. Urgent thrombolysis may be indicated in patients with massive PE obstructing more than 50% of the vasculature. Pulmonary edema and hypotension due to right ventricular failure are consequences of this, and the only way to save such patients may be to remove as much of the obstruction as possible.

▮ 13.5.2 Endovascular Treatment

The purpose of thrombolytic therapy is to reduce the long-term consequences of extensive, particularly caval and iliac DVT. Supposedly it restores patency and preserves valve function but long-term randomized studies comparing this therapy with standard anticoagulation have not been carried out. It may also reveal obstructions contributing to clot formation. Such stenotic segments may be treated by stenting. Thrombolytic therapy achieves more rapid clot resolution but does not significantly reduce mortality or the risk of recurrent PE in hemodynamically stable patients. It is also associated with an increased incidence of major hemorrhage compared with heparin therapy alone. The main contraindications to thrombolysis are listed in Chapter 10 (p. 128).

Therapy should be administered locally by catheter-directed infusion of the lytic agent into the clot. Ipsilateral or contralateral groin access is commonly used. The latter reduces bleeding complications and decreases the risk associated with transversing the thrombus. Thrombus passage increases the risk for clot dislodgement and PE. The ipsilateral approach avoids transversing intact valves, but it may be more difficult to puncture and catheterize the groin vein if it is occluded. Duplex-guided puncture could then be tried. Placing a catheter in the superficial femoral or popliteal veins may be impossible if the valves are intact. A jugular venous catheterization can be used if the clot involves the vena cava. It is common to use a side-hole catheter with its tip placed in the clot.

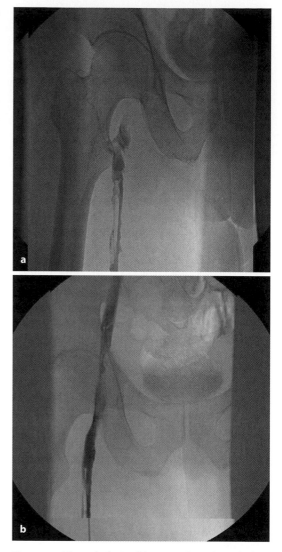

Fig. 13.1. Thrombolysis of iliac vein thrombosis before (**a**) and after therapy (**b**)

When the venous system is catheterized, venography is performed to localize and determine the distribution of the thrombosis. Treatment protocols vary extensively. The first dose of tPA is often infused for 30 min, then the venography is repeated. If more lysis is needed the infusion is continued for 24 h or more. During this time period the result is checked repeatedly, depending on treatment progress. The bolus injection mentioned is not used in some protocols. An example of a venogram is shown in Fig. 13.1.

13.5.3 Operation

Historically, surgical thrombectomy has been liberally used in patients with iliofemoral thrombosis to reduce the risk of postphlebitic syndrome development. Although several patient series have presented good results after thrombectomy, randomized controlled trials data is less favorable. One study reported a similar long-term frequency of postphlebitic syndrome when comparing the procedure with low molecular weight heparin therapy, while others found better preservation of valves and fewer problems after surgery. Considering the general surgical risk and postoperative complications such as groin infection and bleeding, it is rarely indicated to perform surgical venous thrombectomy today. It is used mostly in patients with extensive venous thrombosis who have contraindications for anticoagulation and lytic therapy. Another indication that remains is thrombus extraction in phlegmasia cerulea dolens. The technique of venous thrombectomy is described in the Technical Tips box but can be quite difficult to perform if the experience of vascular surgery is limited.

13.5.4 Phlegmasia Cerulea Dolens

This serious form of DVT is, as already mentioned, characterized by massive thigh and calf edema and a cold, mottled foot. The risk of massive PE is high, even for patients receiving anticoagulation therapy. Phlegmasia cerulea dolens often indicates occult malignancy which must be excluded in every patient.

Treatment follows the principles given for DVT as outlined above, with the addition of fasciotomy when the arterial component is prominent. Thrombolysis is the primary choice when the arterial perfusion is rendered adequate – palpable pulses in the ankle arteries or good skin perfusion in the foot. If the patient lacks foot pulses, surgical thrombectomy is a better strategy because it is a quicker way to reduce clot burden and obstruction. Long-term venous function is of minor importance at this stage. When the arterial function is compromised, fasciotomy should follow the surgical thrombectomy For some patients, amputation is the only option.

TECHNICAL TIPS
Venous Thrombectomy

Preferably, general anesthesia is used and the patient is given an antibiotic that covers common wound infection bacteria. A groin incision is performed right over the common femoral vein, which is extended distally over the superficial femoral vein. These two veins and their branches are exposed and banded. The patient is given intravenous heparin, and a transverse venotomy is performed in the common femoral vein. The anesthesiologist is then asked to adjust the ventilation to a high positive end pressure to minimize the risk of PE, while a #7 or #8 Fogarty catheter is passed proximally into the vena cava and as much of the clot as possible is extracted. This preventive measure is insufficient if the risk for PE is high. If the thrombus protrudes into or involves the vena cava, cava filter insertion should precede surgery. A balloon occluding the vena cava from the contralateral groin could also be used, especially if the thrombus is free floating but located only in the iliac vein. Next, a rubber bandage is tightly applied around the entire leg from the foot to the wound to empty all distal veins from thrombus. Distal thrombectomy can also be done but is often difficult because the valves make distal passage of the Fogarty catheter impossible. Finally, a continuous 5-0 suture closes the venotomy, and an arteriovenous fistula is created. This is achieved by using a branch from the greater saphenous vein and performing an anastomosis between its end and the common femoral artery. The reason for this is that the patency of the iliac vein is considered to be better if a higher flow is achieved. It does require exposure of the artery and its branches. After control of any remaining bleeding, the wound is closed.

■ 13.5.5 Vena Cava Filter Placement

Indications for vena cava filter placement include the following:

- Recurrent PE despite full anticoagulation
- Proximal DVT and contraindications to full anticoagulation
- Proximal DVT and major bleeding while on full anticoagulation
- Progression of iliofemoral clot despite anticoagulation
- Large free-floating thrombus in the iliac vein or inferior vena cava
- Massive PE in which recurrent emboli may prove fatal
- Venous thrombectomy (during or after surgery)

Several types of filters are available on the market, and temporary filters can be used when permanent placement is not necessary; one such situation is the last one in the list above. The complication rate after filter placement is low. Occasionally the filter may be dislodged into the right atrium, but insertion site bleeding is more common. The filter can be inserted by either a jugular or femoral approach. The former is preferred if the CT has revealed extensive thrombus in the inferior vena cava. The method for filter placement via the femoral vein is briefly described in the Technical Tips box.

TECHNICAL TIPS
Vena Cava Filter Placement

Before the procedure it is sometimes necessary to make sure that the iliac veins on the access side and the inferior vena cava are free of thrombus. This is done by cannulating the femoral vein using the Seldinger technique and inserting a guide wire and an introducer sheath. A venogram is obtained by manual injection of contrast. Diameter estimations and better visualization of the vena cava and the renal vein location can be achieved by introducing a pigtail catheter placed higher up. For filter placement, a larger sheath, at least 12-French, is placed over a stiff guide wire approximately to the level where the filter is to be placed. The preloaded filter catheter is advanced to the implant site and released during fluoroscopic monitoring. After the catheter is withdrawn a venogram completes the procedure.

■ 13.5.6 Postoperative Treatment

After thrombolysis or thrombectomy, patients should keep their leg or arm elevated and compression stockings are applied. They should be used day and night for at least 2 weeks postoperatively. Intermittent compression devices increase venous blood flow and probably improve patency after thrombolysis and thrombectomy. For the latter, the benefit is supported by clinical studies. Patients should also receive long-term anticoagulation, initially with low molecular weight heparin that is substituted for coumadin for at least 6 months. If not investigated previously, underlying coagulation disorders should be considered because this would influence the length and type of treatment

■ 13.6 Results and Outcome

There are several studies in the literature comparing thrombolysis and anticoagulation for acute DVT, and meta-analyses suggest that the former is more effective for clot lysis and venous patency. Furthermore, significantly fewer patients appear to end up with postthrombotic syndrome when treated with thrombolysis as compared with anticoagulation. Accordingly, many patients with acute iliofemoral DVT should be considered for thrombolysis. As suspected, however, more bleeding complications occur with this treatment strategy, so careful selection of patients is important. Also, surgical thrombectomy appears to be more effective, than anticoagulation alone. In one study this strategy was able to preserve at least half of the valves and 80% of occluded iliofemoral segments could be reopened.

Few good prospective studies exist on the efficacy of vena cava filters for preventing PE, but at least one randomized controlled trial clearly verified that filters are effective at least in the short term. Accordingly, this study suggests that temporary filters may be advantageous.

13.7 Miscellaneous

13.7.1 Thrombophlebitis

Thrombophlebitis, thrombosis of a superficial vein with secondary inflammation insurrounding tissue, is a very common condition. The exact explanation for its occurrence is unknown, but coagulation disturbances or local inflammation probably contribute. Because varicose veins are prone to be damaged by minor trauma and also often have a low blood flow, they are at risk for thrombophlebitis. Patients with malignancy have an increased risk for this condition and if there are no apparent causes – a known coagulation disorder or trauma – patients should be worked up to rule out other diseases or coagulation problems.

The patient experiences pain in the extremity, which is quite severe and is localized along a superficial vein. The skin feels tender and hot. The physical examination is usually sufficient to reveal the location of the thrombophlebitis as well as its distribution. Because thrombophlebitis in leg veins may spread to the deep system and cause DVT and even PE, it is important to find out whether it extends into deeper veins. In the literature this happens in around 10% of the cases. If one is in doubt, duplex scanning is recommended.

The treatment consists of analgesics, mobilization, and sometimes low molecular weight heparin subcutaneously. The latter is indicated if the patient is unable to walk because of the pain. Thrombophlebitis localized to the thigh, especially close to its inflow into the common femoral vein may be treated by surgical ligation to prevent continued thrombosis in the deep veins and PE. It is common, however, to use a duplex scan to find out the distance from the clot to the common femoral vein. Surgical ligation is recommended if this distance is <1 cm.

Further Reading

Augustinos P, Ouriel K. Invasive approaches to treatment of venous thromboembolism. Circulation 2004; 110(9 Suppl 1):I27–I34

Haage P, Krings T, Schmitz-Rode T. Nontraumatic vascular emergencies: imaging and intervention in acute venous occlusion. Eur Radiol 2002; 12(11):2627–6243

Juhan CM, Alimi YS, Barthelemy PJ, et al. Late results of iliofemoral venous thrombectomy. J Vasc Surg 1997; 25(3):417–422

Plate G, Eklof B, Norgren L, et al. Venous thrombectomy for iliofemoral vein thrombosis – 10 year results of a prospective randomised study. Eur J Vasc Endovasc Surg 1997; 14(5):367–374

Sharafuddin MJ, Sun S, Hoballah JJ, et al. Endovascular management of venous thrombotic and occlusive diseases of the lower extremities. J Vasc Interv Radiol 2003; 14(4):405–423

Watson LI, Armon MP. Thrombolysis for acute deep vein thrombosis. Cochrane Database Syst Rev 2004; 4:CD002783

Acute Problems with Vascular Dialysis Access

14

CONTENTS

■ 14.1 Summary

- Infections in dialysis-access fistulas can cause erosion and lethal bleedings.
- Infections in dialysis accesses should not be debrided in the emergency department.
- The urgency of revision of an occluded access depends on the patient's need for dialysis and on available alternative dialysis options.
- Steal symptoms should be worked up urgently and treated expeditiously.

■ 14.2 Background

A prerequisite for providing hemodialysis to a patient with chronic renal insufficiency is access to a vessel with a good diameter for allowing easy puncture with the large-bore dialysis needles, thus achieving high-volume flow and effective dialysis. This is accomplished by performing vascular access procedures. Two main types of surgically created accesses for hemodialysis exist: autologous arteriovenous (AV) fistulas, usually done at the wrist, and "bridging fistulas" made when a synthetic ePTFE (expanded polytetrafluoroethylene) vascular graft is used as a bridge between an artery and a vein. This latter type will be called an AV graft in this chapter. A common type of bridging fistula is the so-called loop graft, which is tunneled as a loop down the palmar aspect of the forearm, with its inflow and outflow anastomoses in the cubital fossa (Fig.14.1). Straight AV grafts with the inflow at the wrist and outflow in the cubital fossa or in the upper arm are also common. AV fistulas in the upper arm can be created either by keeping the cephalic vein at its location or by superficial transposition of the brachial vein to the

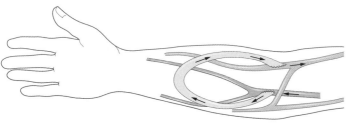

Fig. 14.1. Example of an arterio-venous "loop graft"

volar side of the upper arm. Both alternatives constitute an end-to-side anastomosis to the brachial artery in the cubital fossa. Complications with vascular accesses are a significant problem and cause morbidity as well as mortality in an already severely ill group of patients. The high frequency of complications is reflected in studies from the United States that report at least one urgent reoperation for every third primary operation.

Large numbers of patients need hemodialysis today. In Sweden, for instance, more than 600 patients yearly or at least two patients daily will seek medical attention because of more or less acute problems with their dialysis accesses. The majority will go to hospitals with an established dialysis department and experience managing these complications, but some will be admitted at other institutions for problems related to their dialysis accesses.

Therefore, it is important that most physicians and surgeons are able to recognize complications that need urgent management. The aim of this chapter is to provide a basis for such judgment and to give management recommendations.

14.3 Pathophysiology

The most important acute complications occurring in dialysis accesses and leading to hospital admission are occlusion, infection, bleeding, local swellings, and arterial insufficiency in the hand distal to the access. All complications can occur early after the primary operation or after several years of dialysis. Swelling is usually caused by pseudoaneurysms, hematomas, or seromas. The diagnostic work-up of these complications is in most cases simple, but their management is more difficult. For this reason, the complications will be discussed below under separate headings.

14.3.1 Occlusion and Thrombosis

Early occlusions, up to 4 weeks after access construction, are usually caused by poor preoperative conditions or technical errors at surgery. It is also common, that an AV fistula never develops and matures. This situation can be difficult to differentiate from early thrombosis. Retrospective studies report that 10–25% of all AV fistulas at the wrist level fail to mature.

Late occlusion is caused by a combination of many factors. Dehydration and episodes of hypotension, for example, contribute but are only occasionally the main reason for an occlusion. The significance of stenosis as the cause for occlusion increases over time. Irrespective of access type, stenoses are usually localized in the outflow vein 1–2 cm from the anastomosis. Initially the stenosis causes a resistance against the flow, which decreases it further, and when a critical level is reached the access occludes. Occurrence of multiple stenoses is common for both types of accesses. In AV grafts stenoses are formed both in anastomotic areas and at old puncture sites along the graft itself. The possibilities of a successful thrombectomy are small in late graft occlusions because the risk for multiple stenoses increases with time of usage. Thrombotic occlusion in more proximal segments of the outflow vein, for example at an axillary level, also occurs in a number of cases.

14.3.2 Infection

Between 11% and 35% of all AV grafts will end up with an infectious complication. Postoperative wound infection after access construction belongs to this category and is sometimes related to insufficient skin suturing. Despite intensive antibiotic treatment such infections may spread and form an abscess around the anastomosis. In AV fistulas, infections, other than postoperative ones, are rare; the total infection rate is only 3%. Also, they are often benign and can be treated with antibiotics only. For both access types the infection might erode the walls of the artery or vein with serious bleeding or pseudoaneurysm formation as a consequence.

Even if infections can be fulminant and lead to septicemia and mortality, chronic infections with a more insidious course and mild clinical symptoms are more common. AV grafts are sometimes contaminated at puncture, which causes an infection with few symptoms and a good prognosis. Hematoma development after puncture increases the risk for such infections. They may then be more aggressive, often involving the entire graft with several local abscesses developing along it.

The most common organism found in positive cultures from access infections is Staphylococcus aureus, but streptococci and Gram-negative bacteria are also common. The latter two cause more serious infections than Staphylococcus aureus does.

14.3.3 Bleeding

Bleeding from an AV fistula or graft can occur after trauma or incorrect puncture. A proper technique at puncture is consequently important to avoid unnecessary defects in the graft wall. Even small holes in the fistula vein bleed profusely because of the high flow in the access. It occasionally exceeds 400 ml/min for wrist fistulas and even higher in the upper arm. Infection may also, as already mentioned, lead to disastrous hemorrhage. This is the rationale for a liberal approach to admit the patient for observation when infection in a dialysis access is suspected. Furthermore, the skin covering a dilated vein of an AV fistula is often thin and does not contain bleeding well. Patients with uremia also have a multifactorial disturbance of the coagulation cascade that increases the risk for severe bleeding.

NOTE
Bleeding in well-functioning AV fistulas is often severe due to the high blood flow in the access.

14.3.4 Aneurysms and Hematomas

The reason why some AV fistula veins continue to develop over time to become a true aneurysm is unknown, but the magnitude of blood flow through the access as well as vein quality contribute. Pseudoaneurysms are common in synthetic grafts, secondary to puncture. The frequency is related to the number of punctures in the graft. The incidence is reported to be 10% for AV grafts, while only 2% of AV fistulas are at risk for this complication. As previously mentioned, infection is another important cause of pseudoaneurysm formation that often is located in anastomotic areas.

Hematomas are caused by puncture and are usually absorbed within a couple of weeks. Occasionally a swelling will persist at the hematoma site for a long time. Such swellings consist of fibrosis and serous fluid. Rarely, hematomas become so large that they need surgical treatment.

14.3.5 Steal and Arterial Insufficiency

Steal implies that the blood flow in the graft or fistula is so large that it reduces perfusion to the tissue distal to the fistula. All AV fistulas and grafts cause some degree of steal (Fig. 14.2), but rarely to an extent that symptoms of arterial insufficiency in the hand develop. The frequency of symptomatic arterial insufficiency due to steal is 1–2% for AV fistulas and 5–6% for AV grafts constructed on the forearm. For accesses in the upper arm the frequency is even higher. Patients with diabetes have an increased risk for arterial insufficiency caused by steal.

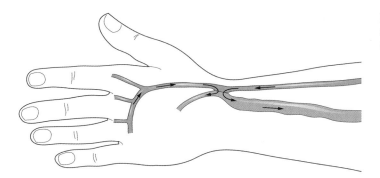

Fig. 14.2. Principle of "steal" in an arteriovenous fistula placed in the wrist

Table 14.1. Medical history in dialysis access occlusion

History	Cause	Management
High resistance during dialysis	Outflow vein stenosis	Revision
"Arterial suction" during dialysis	Inflow artery stenosis	Revision
Puncture difficulties	Impaired access flow (stenosis in the artery)	Revision
Recently constructed access (<4 weeks)	Misjudgment or technical error during operation	Revision
Dehydration	Systemic causes (e.g., gastroenteritis)	Thrombectomy
Episodes of hypotension in association with dialysis	Systemic cause (e.g., medication)	Thrombectomy or thrombolysis
Swollen and discolored hand and arm	Thrombosis/stenosis more proximally in an outflow vein (e.g., external fistula compression during sleep)	New access in the other arm; thrombolysis and angioplasty of stenosis

■ 14.4 Clinical Presentation

Diagnosis of access complications is usually simple. Patients often acquire good knowledge over time about their accesses and are generally well aware of problems. Furthermore, during dialysis two or three times every week the function is evaluated and the fistula examined by nurses. Therefore, the patient is usually admitted with an already established diagnosis. The surgeon's task is then to verify the diagnosis and prepare for treatment.

■ 14.4.1 Occlusions and Thrombosis

The medical history and physical examination are helpful for verifying an occlusion. Some examples from the medical history suggesting different causes for graft occlusion are summarized in Table 14.1.

In AV grafts the function is evaluated by palpation of a thrill and auscultation of bruits over the outflow vein. The thrill feels like a vibration in the fingers. If a thrill is noted and there is an audible bruit, the graft is patent. The direction of flow is sometimes hard to determine in AV grafts. Usually the arterial anastomosis is located on the ulnar side, and the flow is directed in a loop down in the forearm with the venous limb on the radial side (Fig. 14.1). The direction of flow may, however, be the opposite. A simple way to check the flow direction is to occlude the graft at the tip of the loop with a finger and palpate for pulsation over the limbs of the loop. These are then felt only in the arterial limb.

If the access is new and the arm is swollen pulsations can be difficult to find. AV grafts may therefore be patent despite the inability to find a pulse. On the other hand, the graft can be occluded and still have a palpable pulse due to transmission of the pulsation into the thrombus. If, in a previously well-functioning graft, there are neither bruit, thrill, nor pulsations it is occluded.

The examination and evaluation of AV fistulas suspected to be occluded is identical and consists of palpation and auscultation of the outflow vein in search of a thrill and bruit. Pulsations are easier to evaluate in AV fistulas than in AV grafts. AV fistulas can be pulseless and still work well when they are less than 2–3 weeks old. When they have been used for a while they are easy to examine because of the increased vein size. The occurrence of new pulsations in an old fistula indicates a minor outflow obstruction. Total absence of pulses in a vein with previous pulsations strongly indicates occlusion. One alternative for evaluating the patency of an AV fistula is to carefully compress the outflow vein somewhat in the cubital fossa or axilla (for upper arm fistulas) and then search for pulsations.

14.4.2 Other Complications

The clinical presentation of access infections is in line with infectious complications in general, and the patient describes pain, tenderness, fever, and drainage of pus. The severity of the infection should also be assessed because it leads management. Serious infection is associated with septicemia and bleeding and may need urgent management, whereas mild infections can be observed. Early after surgery for AV graft construction the skin may be red and the surgical area swollen. Such findings in the examination suggest a reaction to the graft material, and it usually dissolves within 3–4 days. It is important to also evaluate the function of the fistula and graft because infection may cause and be a consequence of occlusion. When taking a medical history from a patient with a bleeding complication, questions about infection symptoms should be included. It is also important to note signs of infection during the examination of swellings and hematomas. A pulsating mass indicates presence of an aneurysm. If such a pulsating mass is located in the anastomotic area, the aneurysm probably originates from the suture line.

Patients with steal complain about pain, numbness, coldness, and weakness in the hand distal to the access. The symptoms are often accentuated during dialysis. As for atherosclerotic arm ischemia, the patient may have aggravated symptoms when using the hand in an elevated position. The examination may reveal necrotic tips of the fingers, pallor, and cyanosis, and only a weak radial pulse is palpated. Sometimes the pulse is totally absent.

NOTE

Steal may cause severe ischemic problems and should be worked up and treated promptly.

14.5 Diagnostics

Only a few cases of access complications need immediate treatment. These urgent cases need no diagnostic work-up besides the medical history and a physical examination. The cornerstone of the work-up of dialysis access complications is otherwise duplex scanning. Diagnoses of aneurysms and hematomas as well as evaluation of steal and arterial insufficiency generally require duplex. Duplex also provides sufficient information for treatment planning. There is no urgency in working up these complications, and there is always time for a duplex investigation. For symptomatic steal, angiography is used by some as the first choice because of its capability to provide a view of the retrograde and collateral blood flow. In AV graft and fistula thrombosis, diagnostic work-up is rarely necessary. Accesses with poor function are best treated before they occlude. Accordingly, if a problematic access is still patent when examined, duplex should be performed liberally as soon as possible to localize stenoses and provide a revision strategy. Angiography is an alternative if duplex is not available.

14.6 Management and Treatment

14.6.1 Occlusion and Thrombosis

14.6.1.1 In the Emergency Department

Acute occlusion of a hemodialysis access is not a vascular emergency. The only possible exception to this principle is when a recently created AV fistula occludes. After just 6–8 h the thrombus destroys the intima of the vein and the access cannot be salvaged. Accordingly, recent occlusions may be treated by thrombectomy and revision. For occlusions of longer duration little can be done to save the fistula and the main concern is the patient's uremia and urgency of dialysis. As soon as possible a strategy for continued access and dialysis should be formed in collaboration with the nephrologist. The following questions need to be considered to decide whether thrombectomy or thrombolysis should be attempted:

- Has this access had previous problems and been revised before?
- What is the chance that the access can be used for dialysis after thrombectomy and revision?
- Which alternative access routes are available?

If the access has had problems and been revised previously and there is little chance that dialysis can be continued it is often better to consider the alternatives to thrombectomy. When few access possibilities are available it is reasonable to be more aggressive with thrombectomy attempts.

AV grafts, on the other hand, can more often be saved by thrombectomy or thrombolysis. We recommend doing the operation as soon as possible, but not during nighttime. Thrombolysis is a good alternative for AV graft occlusions.

14.6.1.2 Operation

A surgeon without experience in access surgery is almost never forced to perform an operation without being able to wait for assistance. The only possible exception to this is thrombectomy. Therefore, in this text only this procedure will be described in detail and other operations will be discussed in more general terms. The technique is described in the Technical Tips box. It must be remembered, however, that simple thrombectomy as the only procedure is rarely successful; it is primarily recommended in cases when an anatomical cause for the occlusion has been ruled out. It usually has to be combined with some kind of revision.

TECHNICAL TIPS
Thrombectomy in an AV Fistula

Local or regional anesthesia of the axillary plexus is preferred, but if an increased risk of bleeding is reported, it should be avoided. Protection masks and double gloves should be used because of the hepatitis risk. Scrub and drape the entire arm. For correction of AV fistulas, a longitudinal incision at least 5 cm long over the outflow vein is recommended. The distal end of the incision should be placed at the level of the anastomosis. The fistula is exposed by sharp dissection and a vessel loop is applied. At this stage the fistula is checked again for patency by palpation or a pen Doppler. The vein is then inspected for the presence of stenoses, which are seen as a narrowing combined with a poststenotic dilatation (Fig. 14.3). The stenotic area can also be palpated as a segment with a thick and hard vessel wall. A transverse incision is made in the vein as close to the anastomosis as possible. Thrombectomy in the outflow vein is performed first in a proximal direction toward the upper arm using a #3 Fogarty catheter until no further thrombus material comes out through the venotomy. If backflow is restored, vein function is checked once more by rapidly infusing heparinized Ringer's glucose solution. Infusion of 20 ml should be easily done within 20–30 s with no resistance. If a large force is required, remaining thrombus or stenoses in the outflow or axillary vein is probable. The best way to verify this is to perform an intraoperative angiography and this is recommended when there is any uncertainty about the results. When venous outflow is restored, the vein is clamped with a small soft vascular clamp such as a mini-bulldog. At this stage systemic heparinization is considered; the recommended dose is half the normal dose of 50–75 units heparin per kilogram of body weight. The next step is to insert the same thrombectomy catheter toward the inflow anastomosis and into the artery. One pull with the catheter is usually enough to obtain a strong pulsating inflow. Finally, the vessel is clamped and the venotomy closed with interrupted 6-0 or 7-0 prolene sutures. The result is evaluated by palpating the vein and auscultating with a pen Doppler. If the pulse and Doppler signals are weak, it is necessary to continue the operation with revision of the access.

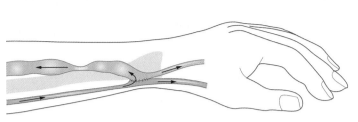

Fig. 14.3. Stenosis in an arteriovenous fistula

AV grafts

The technique for thrombectomy of thrombosed AV grafts and fistulas is the same. Synthetic grafts are more prone to infection and antibiotic prophylaxis is recommended. The easiest way to expose the graft is at the tip of the loop or in the midportion of a straight graft. It is better to make the skin incision parallel and lateral to the graft then over it. A transverse incision increases the risk of incision complications such as tissue necrosis and graft infection. Alternatively, the incision can be placed in the old scar from the primary operation over the venous anastomosis. This is favorable when there is a history of malfunction that suggests a possible outflow stenosis. The dissection to expose AV grafts is sometimes cumbersome because of the extensive fibrosis that evolves after implantation. Careless dissection can create holes in the graft that will cause problems when flow is restored. An example is extensive pulling of the graft to facilitate dissection. Bleeding from holes in the graft some distance from the skin incision is best controlled by a #4 Fogarty catheter inflated and closed with a three-way stopcock. The graft should be controlled using a molded vascular clamp to avoid mechanical damage to the graft. Otherwise, the description in the Technical Tips box for thrombectomy of AV fistulas is also valid for AV grafts.

Revision

The purpose of revision is to correct the problem that has caused the occlusion of the access or threatens its function. Stenosed segments in an AV fistula or graft are replaced with a vein or PTFE interposition graft. Patching of the stenosed area enlarges an anastomosis that is stenosed. Sometimes both interposition grafting and patch repair need to be done. Alternatives at revision are to move the outflow anastomosis to a more proximal location on the same vein or switch it to a different outflow vein.

14.6.1.3 Thrombolysis

Thrombolysis is an alternative to thrombectomy. It has the advantage of avoiding surgery and general anesthesia, and central stenoses contributing to access occlusion can be corrected by angioplasty. Such proximal lesions are harder to treat by open surgery. It is a matter of debate whether thrombolysis should be performed instead of thrombectomy and revision. Patients with contraindications to thrombolysis are not candidates, but for other groups the literature is contradictory. Thrombolysis is certainly feasible, but recent data suggest a slight advantage for the open procedure in terms of outcome. In some hospitals, thrombolysis is attempted with a few days' delay to reduce the risk of bleeding after a failed thrombectomy.

The thrombolytic procedure of AV grafts usually involves catheterizing the graft where it is easy to puncture. For loop grafts the tip is one such site. A guide wire is introduced into the venous limb first, which is then substituted for a pulse spray catheter via a 4-French dilator. The tip should initially be placed well into the outflow vein to enable venography to rule out central stenoses. After the tip is placed within the thrombus, a separate puncture is performed to catheterize the arterial limb in a similar way. After local heparinization thrombolysis is initiated through both catheters. Thrombolysis of AV fistulas is more difficult and the outcome cumbersome. Entrance to a fistulas is achieved as close as possible to the anastomosis and a venogram is obtained to visualize the branches of the open vein. An end-hole catheter is often used and the bolus injection omitted.

14.6.2 Infections

14.6.2.1 In the Emergency Department

Patients with suspected access-area infections should be admitted for observation unless the clinical presentation indicates a localized mild infection. Wounds should not be debrided in the emergency department because it might cause profuse bleeding. Instead, the wound should be cleansed and dressed with pads containing an antiseptic solution, and antibiotics covering Staphylococcus aureus should be prescribed. Before antibiotics are administered samples for microbiological culture should be gathered. If possible, the arm should be kept elevated to decrease swelling.

When more severe infection is suspected, parenteral antibiotics are recommended. If a local infection of an AV graft is complicated by septicemia the graft must be extirpated immediately. A patient with septicemia on dialysis without signs of infection over the access can be treated with antibiotics for a couple of days before extirpation is considered.

14.6.2.2 Operation

AV graft removal under local anesthesia should be avoided because exposure of the entire anastomotic area is necessary, and sufficient analgesia is hard to achieve in infectious tissue. The skin incision is placed in the old scar from the primary operation. Occasionally, the graft is not incorporated and surrounded with pus and fluid and can easily be pulled out of its subcutaneous channel. Further incisions along the graft are often needed to expose and enable excision of the entire graft. Graft extirpation necessitates control of all inflow and outflow vessels with vascular clamps. After the total graft is removed the arteriotomy is closed using an autologous vein patch. Direct suture of the arterial defect should be avoided because of risk for arterial narrowing and tension in the suture line, thus increasing the risk for continued infection and bleeding. The vein can be ligated. The brachial artery may also be ligated when the dissection to expose the arterial anastomosis is very difficult. Usually the collateral circulation is sufficient. In such difficult situations an alternative when the graft is well incorporated in the area around the arterial anastomosis, is to leave a 5-mm-long cuff and oversew it. This is, however, associated with a much higher risk for continued infection and reoperation. During surgery samples for microbiological cultures are obtained from pus or fluid in the graft tunnel. If the infection appears to be very local, as when contaminated by puncture, the access may be saved by interposition of a new piece of graft tunneled through an area without infection.

An infected AV fistula is ligated on the inflow side at least 1 cm away from the infected area to avoid bleeding. A new access should not be constructed until the infection is completely healed.

14.6.3 Bleeding

14.6.3.1 In the Emergency Department

As for all major bleeding, the wound should be manually compressed immediately. If bleeding continues and is profuse the patient should be taken to the operating room for exploration and control. When finger compression is insufficient to control the bleeding, a tourniquet can be used. It is placed in the upper arm and inflated to a pressure 50 mmHg over the systolic blood pressure. To avoid damage to the skin the cuff should be padded. As soon as the bleeding site is surgically exposed and controlled the tourniquet is deflated. In cases of major bleeding an intravenous line is placed for blood sampling and volume replacement.

For minor bleedings, such as from a puncture site, the patient is admitted for continuing compression and monitoring. Digital compression is maintained for 20–30 min because it enables adequate compression without obstructing the graft or fistula flow. If the bleeding has stopped after this time, digital compression can be substituted with a compression bandage. If bleeding continues despite several hours of compression, the patient should be worked up for a potential coagulation disorder. Pharmacological treatment should be started after considering the risk of graft thrombosis. Surgical repair of minor hemorrhage should be avoided as much as possible. Rarely the source is surgical, and control and repair often necessitate a fairly extensive procedure.

14.6.3.2 Operation

The basic principle for surgical repair of bleeding from holes in AV grafts and fistulas is to obtain proximal and distal control through incisions in intact skin and excise and replace the injured segment with an interposition graft. This is favored over suturing the hole with or without a patch. The latter is more difficult and often causes a narrowing and increases the risk of postoperative thrombosis. For large amounts of bleeding, the procedure can be performed in a bloodless field obtained by tourniquet occlusion.

14.6.4 Aneurysms and Hematomas

14.6.4.1 In the Emergency Department
Patients with a thin skin layer covering a clinically suspected aneurysm are at risk for fistula rupture. These aneurysms should therefore be subject to surgical excision. Urgent management is particularly important when there are signs of infection because such aneurysms may cause septic embolization in addition to severe bleeding. The patient needs urgent work-up with duplex scanning to differentiate such infected aneurysms from other fluid collections that do not need urgent management.

Hematomas that not are infected are best left to reabsorb. Exceptions are hematomas that compress the access and might impair its flow. Duplex is helpful for evaluating whether this is the case. If the hematoma is expanding rapidly, within a couple of hours, blood flow in the access is almost always threatened. Such expansion is usually caused by graft laceration and should be immediately repaired. Old and stable hematomas can, as an alternative, be treated by puncture and aspiration if the function of the access is at risk. To avoid infection the puncture should be performed as far away from the graft as possible.

14.6.4.2 Operation
True aneurysms with an overlying skin defect in AV fistulas are excised after proximal and distal control. Venous interposition grafting repairs the defect. Surgical treatment of pseudoaneurysms in AV grafts also requires control proximal and distal to the aneurysm. The aneurysm is then opened and the connection between the sac and graft lumen is oversewn. Resection and interposition of a new piece of graft is often required, however. In the anastomotic area, pseudoaneurysms are best excised and the defect repaired with a patch. A hematoma threatening the graft's function is treated the same way as aneurysms.

14.6.4 Arterial Insufficiency and Steal

14.6.4.1 In the Emergency Department
Arterial insufficiency secondary to steal is not managed urgently. Diagnostic work-up with duplex or angiography is usually necessary to plan an adequate treatment strategy. Administration of analgesics should be initiated as soon as possible, and opioids are often required. Even in patients with severe ischemic symptoms, ligature of grafts or fistulas can be performed during office hours. Occasional patients with therapy-resistant pain might need urgent surgery.

14.6.4.2 Operation
In patients with severe symptoms of hand ischemia the AV fistula or graft must be closed. This is achieved by exposing the vein in the anastomotic area and clamping the artery. The vein is then divided and closed by sutures 1 or 2 cm from the anastomosis. Upper arm AV fistulas are treated the same way. Attempts to reduce blood flow at this level by wrapping a vein or synthetic patch around the fistula have anecdotally been successful. Occasionally, work-up of arterial insufficiency caused by AV fistulas in the wrist reveals retrograde flow in the hand. These patients can sometimes be improved by simply transforming the anastomosis from side-by-side to end-by-side. Usually, however, ligation of the entire fistula is required.

AV grafts causing steal are excised as described in the section on infection, but the access may be saved by using a different technique. It constitutes a bypass from the brachial artery above the inflow anastomosis to a level below it. The bypass is then followed by ligature of the brachial artery just distal to the proximal bypass anastomosis. With this method relief of ischemic symptoms with maintained access function has been reported.

14.6.5 Management After Treatment

The principles for management after treatment are similar for all complication types. Surgical wounds should be inspected frequently during the first 24 h. Bleeding problems are common after thrombectomy and revision as well as after procedures for infection and steal. Function is also monitored closely. Patency is checked by auscultating for bruits and palpating for thrills over the outflow vein. After AV graft procedures, the vein is insonated at the vein and graft anastomosis site.

It is important to ensure that the patient is hydrated and has an acceptable blood pressure. This is often a difficult task in uremic patients. If a stenosis is suspected in the access but is not mended for some reason, a duplex scan is ordered as soon as possible to verify and localize it before the access reoccludes. Postoperative heparinization beyond the dialysis treatment is rarely needed. Patients treated for infection should continue on antibiotics until the results of bacterial cultures arrive or the infection is healed.

14.6.6 When Can the Patient be Given Dialysis?

For all problems with dialysis accesses an important issue is the patient's need for dialysis. Inserting a temporary catheter in the neck or groin should be weighed against the possibility of a successful operation. A basic rule is that a revised dialysis access should be allowed at least a couple of days to heal after the procedure to avoid bleeding complications. Dialysis requires heparinization, which in combination with uremic patients' tendency for coagulopathy increases the risk for bleeding. During dialysis clots in the suture line are dissolved and bleeding is likely. Such bleeding is often difficult to treat. Moreover, interposed vein grafts have thin walls and are easy to damage during puncture. Vein grafts needs at least 10–14 days to be arterialized, and PTFE grafts should be incorporated in surrounding tissue to minimize the risk for bleeding. Accordingly, if the need for dialysis is urgent and the risk of surgical bleeding after revision is considered small, dialysis can be performed the first postoperative day providing that the puncture can be made in an old part of the access and that the heparin dose during dialysis is adjusted.

14.7 Results and Outcome

In Sweden AV fistulas constitute about 80% of all dialysis accesses constructed. This percentage varies internationally, but the trend is that AV fis-

Table 14.2. Location of stenosis in 357 arteriovenous grafts[a] (based on four studies)

Localization	Frequency
Venous anastomosis	63%
In vein away from the anastomosis	18%
In inflow artery	10%
In graft	12%
In a central vein	1%

[a] 36% had more than one localization

tulas are preferred over AV grafts. The reason is that if an AV fistula develops – which about 75% does – it will probably work well for many years with few complications. Compared with AV grafts stenoses in the outflow vein develop later in AV fistulas; the mean difference is in the range of 4–5 months. AV grafts, however, have the advantage of early dialysis, and at least 70% of all grafts are patent one year after implantation. Later AV grafts are prone to develop stenoses and infection complicates this type of access in much higher frequencies. The locations of stenoses in AV grafts are listed in Table 14.2.

The result of thrombectomy for treatment access occlusion is poor. For example, one study evaluating AV grafts reported a 75% immediate success, but the 30-day patency was 45%. At 6 months only 18% of the grafts could be used for dialysis and at 1 year only 3% could. A contributing factor to these results is probably that some stenoses are missed at thrombectomy and are not corrected. This is supported in the literature, which reports that half of all occluded AV grafts have no identifiable cause of occlusion. When angiography was performed in the same patient group, 92% had at least one stenosis. When thrombectomy was combined with revision the results were somewhat better: 60% of the grafts were patent after 30 days and 25% at 6 months. In most studies, multiple revisions are often needed to achieve acceptable results. Only a few AV fistulas can be saved by thrombectomy according to the literature, which is why this operation should not be performed often. It is generally better to create a new access if the occlusion lasts longer than 8 h and when the fistula occludes early after construction.

Further Reading

Bush RL, Lin PH, Lumsden AB. Management of thrombosed dialysis access: thrombectomy versus thrombolysis. Semin Vasc Surg 2004; 17(1):32–39

Green LD, Lee DS, Kucey DS. A metaanalysis comparing surgical thrombectomy, mechanical thrombectomy, and pharmacomechanical thrombolysis for thrombosed dialysis grafts. J Vasc Surg 2002; 36(5):939–945

Huber TS, Buhler AG, Seeger JM. Evidence-based data for the hemodialysis access surgeon. Semin Dial 2004; 17(3):217–223

Lew SQ, Kaveh K. Dialysis access related infections. ASAIO J 2000; 46(6):S6–S12

Schanzer H, Eisenberg D. Management of steal syndrome resulting from dialysis access. Semin Vasc Surg 2004; 17(1):45–49

Tordoir JH, Dammers R, van der Sande FM. Upper extremity ischemia and hemodialysis vascular access. Eur J Vasc Endovasc Surg 2004; 27(1):1–5

General Principles of Vascular Surgical Technique **15**

CONTENTS

■ 15.1 Summary

- Always use atraumatic technique and special vascular instruments.
- For proximal and distal control, all inflow and outflow vessels must be controlled and clamped prior to repair or arteriotomy or venotomy.
- Blind application of vascular clamps in a bleeding traumatic wound as dangerous.
- A nonsecure distal intimal edge is always a risk for dissection and creation of an intimal flap causing occlusion.
- Veins are vulnerable and extreme care is necessary during dissection and repair.
- A vascular suture should always be tied with the artery clamped.

■ 15.2 Background

For surgeons who do not routinely perform vascular operations it might be helpful to recapitulate the basic vascular surgical technique to facilitate their management of common vascular emergencies. First, it is always necessary to obtain control of and clamp all branches to the of interest vascular segment to make a vascular operation possible at all. The rationale for being extra cautious with blood vessels is that they are extremely sensitive to trauma, which can induce undesired thrombogenic activity on the intimal surface. Furthermore, their structure of separated wall layers demands special consideration to avoid dissection and occlusion. A successful vascular operation requires the surgeon to pay constant attention to technical details to avoid jeopardizing the entire operation.

■ 15.3 Exposure

Good exposure is always mandatory for optimizing the prerequisites for reconstruction or repair. Exposure of most specific vascular segments is described in the corresponding chapter (e.g., exposure of the superficial femoral artery in the groin for embolectomy is covered in the chapter on acute leg ischemia).

With a few exceptions (for instance, the transverse incision in the cubital fossa for exposing the brachial artery), a longitudinal skin incision over the vessel is used. The incision is made approximately 2 cm longer in each direction than the required exposed vessel length. An incision that is too small increases the risk for wound complications in the skin and other tissues with already impaired perfusion due to unnecessary trauma from retractors. Familiarity with the anatomy is essential because it is not always possible to be guided by palpation of a pulse or hard arteriosclerotic plaques. Use small, blunt, self-retaining retractors to achieve tension in the tissue to facilitate dissection. When approaching the vessel special atraumatic vascular instruments should always be used. Never use a toothed forceps in the vicinity of a blood vessel. The correct plane of final exposure is the outer soft layer of the adventitia. A common error is exaggerated caution in trying to obtain exposure in a layer that is too superficial. The adventitia is characterized by a visible net of vasa vasorum. It is important to be aware of the differences between a healthy and a diseased artery. The former is soft, easily compressible, and has a grey/red color. This is what can be expected in trauma patients who are mostly young and otherwise healthy. When there is no pulse in the artery it may even be difficult to distinguish it from a vein. An arteriosclerotic artery in a patient with peripheral vascular disease is yellow/white and has a thick and often hard or calcified wall.

Expose the anterior and lateral aspects of the artery and use a right-angle clamp with its tip turned away from the adjacent larger vein – thus avoiding accidental perforations – to surround the posterior aspect with a vessel-loop of fabric or rubber. By lifting the vessel-loop, tension can be achieved in the tissue, thus facilitating the dissection in an atraumatic way (Fig. 15.1). All branches should be saved because they are potential important collaterals.

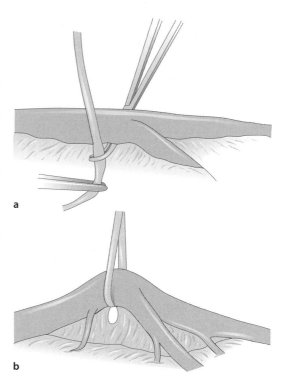

a

b

Fig. 15.1. a Pass a right-angle clamp gently through the soft tissue on the dorsal aspect of the artery and direct it away from larger veins to avoid iatrogenic injuries. Caution! Avoid accidental penetration of the dorsal wall of the artery. **b** Gently lift the artery with the vessel-loop to achieve tension in the tissue, thus facilitating the dissection

NOTE

> **Good exposure of the segment to be repaired, including space enough to allow safe clamping, is essential for a successful vascular operation. Always use special atraumatic vascular instruments when approaching the vessel.**

■ 15.4 Control of Bleeding and Clamping

In all vascular procedures, including vascular trauma, proximal and distal control is mandatory before attempting repair or doing an arteriotomy. It is desirable to have a completely empty vascular segment in order to perform a vascular operation without unnecessary technical difficulties. To

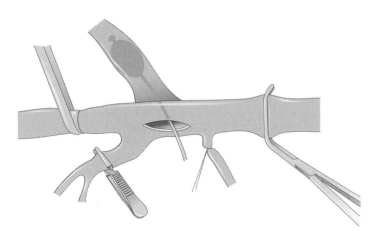

Fig. 15.2. Different methods for controlling bleeding are demonstrated. From left to right: doubly applied vessel-loop, "bulldog" (small metallic vascular clamp), balloon catheter, loop of ligature, vascular clamp

achieve this, all branches for inflow as well as outflow from the segment must be controlled. Before clamping, systemic anticoagulation is usually necessary unless contraindicated by bleeding risk. The standard dose is 100 units/kg body weight of heparin given intravenously, but in practice, 5,000 units is usually adequate for an adult patient. It is important to be aware that the activity of heparin is halved within 1–2 h, so a repeated dose of 2,500 units might be required, especially if the surgeon notices increased clotting activity in the operating field. For local heparinization, flushing with a solution of 5,000 units of heparin in 500 ml Ringer's acetate or Ringer's glucose (10 units/ml) is recommended.

Control of the flow in the exposed vascular segments is achieved with different types of vascular clamps or with vessel-loops of cotton fabric or rubber. Doubly applied 2-0 or 3-0 ligatures can also be used for smaller branches. Intraluminal control with balloon catheters can also be effective (Fig. 15.2).

A vascular clamp should be chosen with an angle and shape that minimally disturbs the surgical exposure during the rest of the procedure. To avoid disrupting the often dorsally located plaques in arteriosclerotic arteries, clamps should preferably be applied horizontally and closed just enough to stop the blood flow (Fig. 15.3).

Temporary vascular clamps can be manufactured using vessel-loops or umbilical tape and a piece of rubber tubing (Fig. 15.4).

When there is active traumatic bleeding, a blindly applied vascular clamp can be dangerous and should be avoided. For full control, the injured vascular segment must be exposed. The bleeding vessel can be controlled by finger compression, a "peanut," or a "strawberry" until the vessel has been mobilized and the bleeding controlled. If this technique is not possible, external compression and packing of the wound with dressings under compression can be used while dissection is performed and adequate exposure obtained, but this usually results in significant blood loss.

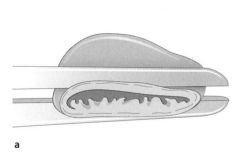

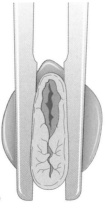

Fig. 15.3. Arteriosclerotic plaques are usually located dorsally in the artery. The clamp should be placed horizontally to avoid plaque fracture and fragmentation

a

b

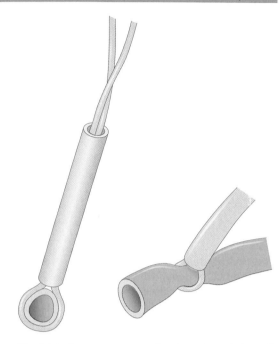

Fig. 15.4. A temporary vascular clamp is made by pulling a double vessel-loop through a piece of rubber tubing to make a snare around the vessel, which is locked by an ordinary clamp

In certain situations, such as in scar tissue, thorough dissection of a vascular segment can be technically very challenging and should thus be avoided. Balloon occlusion can be a very good alternative for distal as well as temporary proximal control. Control is, however, best achieved by surgical exposure and clamping of a more proximal segment, while balloon occlusion is always an alternative for distal control. Embolectomy catheters of adequate size connected to a three-way stopcock and a saline-filled syringe are used. Inspection of the open segment, under continuous evacuation of blood from the backbleeding branches with suction, allows identification of the orifice into which the catheter should be inserted. After insertion the balloon is insufflated until the backflow has ceased. The stopcock is closed, and the balloon is left in place to occlude the artery. It is important not to overinflate the balloon, which could damage the arterial wall. In analogy with a vascular clamp, the balloon should be insufflated just to the point when bleeding stops – no further.

In larger arteries such as the aorta, a Foley catheter of appropriate size can be used for the same purpose. Special catheters from different manufacturers are also available for occluding arteries. When balloons are used for proximal control they are easily dislocated and even blown out by the arterial pressure. This can be avoided by having an assistant manually support the catheter or by applying a vascular tape around the artery just proximal to the arteriotomy, thus preventing the balloon from being further dislocated distally.

NOTE

Never open a blood vessel without having proximal and distal control.

■ 15.4.1 Proximal Endovascular Aortic Control

When available, this alternative is of great potential importance for patients with severe intraabdominal bleeding after rupture of aneurysms as well as traumatic vascular injuries. It is further described in Chapter 7 (p. 85).

■ 15.5 Vascular Suture

When vessels are sutured, the suture should include all the layers of the vessel wall. The adventitia is the most important layer for the mechanical strength of the vascular wall. The adventitia should not be allowed to be interposed between the approximated edges of the arteriotomy because that can disturb the healing process. This can be avoided by everting the edges to allow intima-to-intima approximation.

When vessels are being sutured, the needle's point should be placed at a 90° angle against the vascular wall, and thereafter its circular shape is used to push it through the wall to avoid unnecessary tearing. It is important to place the needle from inside out, particularly on the downstream side of the vascular suture, in order to fasten and secure the intima, avoid splitting the wall layers, and avoid the risk of intimal dissection (Fig. 15.5).

Arteriosclerotic arteries can be very hard and calcified, making penetration of the needle at an ideal site impossible. In such a situation it might

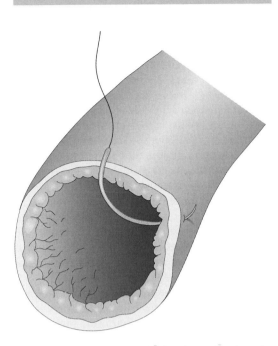

Fig. 15.5. The needle should be directed 90° to the vessel wall. Always include the intima, especially on the downstream side, to avoid dissection of the distal intimal edge

be necessary to penetrate the vascular wall with the needle and suture at a far distance from the intended suture row. Sometimes it is necessary to remove an extensive and hard arteriosclerotic plaque by a local thrombendarterectomy before the repair can be completed. Another important detail in suturing arteries is to tighten the suture satisfactorily; a suture that is too loose will cause leakage, and if it is too tight this will certainly lead to stenosis. The angle when pulling the suture should be 90° from the vascular wall to minimize the risk of tears in the vascular wall. Oozing in the suture row is best managed by tamponade with a sponge for 5–10 min or until bleeding stops. If extra hemostatic sutures are needed, a suture one size smaller than those in the suture row is recommended. If the result is unsatisfactory a local hemostatic agent can be applied.

Simple suturing for minor traumatic injuries in arteries is demonstrated in Fig. 15.6. It is important to tie the suture with the artery clamped and not pulsating to get it properly adjusted.

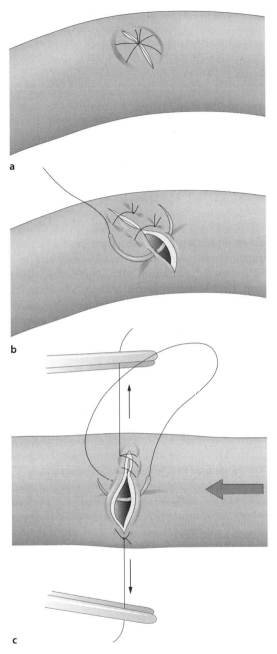

Fig. 15.6. **a** Simple cross-suture of an arterial puncture. **b** Simple sutures in a transverse arterial injury or arteriotomy. **c** If the artery is large (>10 mm wide) a running suture can be used

15.5.1 Choice of Suture Material

Vascular sutures are monofilament, synthetic, and double-armed. The needles are taper-pointed and have a variety of curvatures. Most vascular needles are larger than the suture to which they are attached. This can be a source of suture-line bleeding, which is best treated with local compression and hemostatic agents, but not with further sutures. Recommendations for sutures are given in Table 15.1 below.

Table 15.1. Suture sizes for various vessel segments

Vessel	Suture size
Aorta	3-0 to 4-0
Iliac arteries	5-0
Femoral artery	5-0
Popliteal above the knee	5-0 or 6-0
Popliteal below the knee	6-0
Calf artery	6-0 or 7-0
Carotid	6-0
Brachial	6-0
Subclavian	5-0
Renal – visceral	6-0

15.6 Arteriotomy

When performing an arteriotomy it is important to avoid damaging the vessel's posterior wall, to choose the right direction of arteriotomy, and to close it properly. An arteriotomy starts with puncture with a pointed scalpel blade (#11) with the edge turned away from the surgeon. When a puncture bleeding is obtained, the blade is moved forward and upward to avoid injuries to the posterior wall. The lower blade of a 60° vascular scissors (Pott's scissors) is inserted into the arteriotomy, which is elongated appropriately while ensuring that the scissors is in the true free vascular lumen and not within any of the layers of the vascular wall. Because arteriosclerotic arteries are occasionally extremely hard, the best site for arteriotomy is chosen by palpating with a finger to find a soft segment. Choosing the arteriotomy direction, transverse or longitudinal, is sometimes difficult and is worth special consideration.

Longitudinal arteriotomy is the most useful and has the advantage of being easily elongated. It allows better inspection of the vascular lumen and can be used for an end-to-side anastomosis if reconstruction is necessary. On the other hand, it must be closed with a patch to avoid narrowing of arteries with a diameter <5 mm (see below).

Transverse arteriotomy can be considered when the procedure is likely to be limited to an embolectomy and when the artery is thinner than 5 mm. When closing the arteriotomy, it is always important to start by catching the intima with the needle at the distal end of the arteriotomy to avoid dissection and occlusion. A running suture is mainly used (Fig. 15.7), but in transverse arteriotomies in smaller arteries, simple sutures are preferable to avoid the risk of narrowing by a running suture that is too tight.

15.7 Closure with Patch (Patch Angioplasty)

The patch technique is very important and useful in all emergency vascular procedures. A patch should always be considered when closing an artery after longitudinal arteriotomy or traumatic injury with a vessel wall defect. A longitudinal suture always causes a certain degree of narrowing because the suture needle is placed 1–2 mm from the edge on both sides. A basic rule is that vessels

Fig. 15.7. Closure of a longitudinal arteriotomy with a running suture

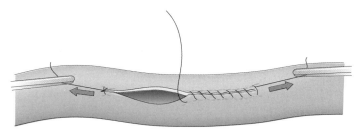

with diameters <5 mm should be closed with a patch. Occasionally, even larger arteries should be closed by the patch technique. In practice, patches are frequently used for the calf, popliteal, brachial, carotid, and sometimes also the femoral and iliac arteries. The choice of patch material depends on location and the level of contamination. An autologous vein is recommended in the superficial femoral artery and distally. In the common femoral artery, iliac arteries, and the aorta, a synthetic polyester or polytetrafluoroethylene (PTFE) graft is most commonly used.

The patch technique is demonstrated in Fig. 15.8. The patch should be cut to an appropriate width, aiming to compensate for the diameter loss but with some oversizing. Too large a patch will cause a disadvantageous enlargement, which subsequently might lead to increased risk for development of aneurysms and thrombotic occlusions. The patch is shaped at the end in a rounded fashion. The suture is started at one of the ends, possibly with retaining sutures in both ends. It is always important to ensure that the distal intimal edge is secured by the suture. The suture is tied in the middle of the patch and never at one of the ends.

NOTE
Always consider using a patch when closing vessels <5 mm in diameter.

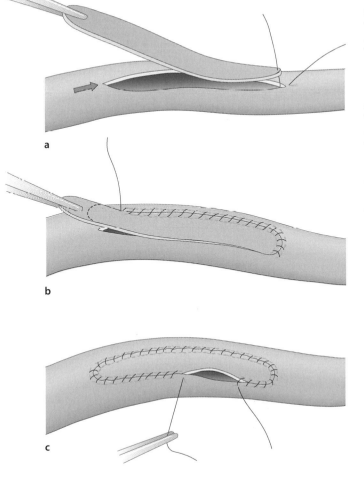

Fig. 15.8. Patch closure of a longitudinal arteriotomy. **a** The suture is started distally (downstream) with the needle from inside to out to secure the distal intima. The first suture can be tied to secure the patch before proceeding with the suture row. **b** The suture is continued in a running fashion in both directions and always with the needle running from the inside to the outside of the artery. When the proximal end of the arteriotomy is approached, the patch has to be cut and trimmed. **c** The sutures are continued until they meet on one of the sides. Check inflow and backflow before tying

■ 15.8 Interposition Graft

To bridge a defect in an artery a piece of a vascular graft is interponated. A vein graft is used for the arms and infrainguinally in the legs. In larger arteries including the iliac arteries and the aorta, a synthetic prosthesis can be used. If the vessels that are going to be anastomosed end to end have different diameters, the ends should be cut obliquely to adjust the circumference of both ends to each other. After transverse resection of the thinner vessel, its end is cut longitudinally and the corners trimmed. The larger vessel also needs to be cut

slightly transversally to avoid kinking in the anastomosis (Fig. 15.9). Also, when thinner vessels are going to be anastomosed end to end, the circumference and width of the anastomosis must be ensured by cutting both ends obliquely. This will minimize the risk for narrowing in the suture row.

If the anastomosis is started by two diametrically opposite holding sutures, the suture adjustment is facilitated and the posterior aspect can easily be rotated with the two holding sutures. The anastomosis is then completed with a running suture of appropriate size (Fig. 15.10). As pointed out

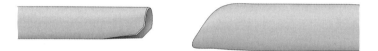

Fig. 15.9. When two vessels with different diameters are being sutured end to end, the smaller has to be slit open and the edges trimmed to fit the larger one, which must be cut somewhat obliquely to avoid kinking

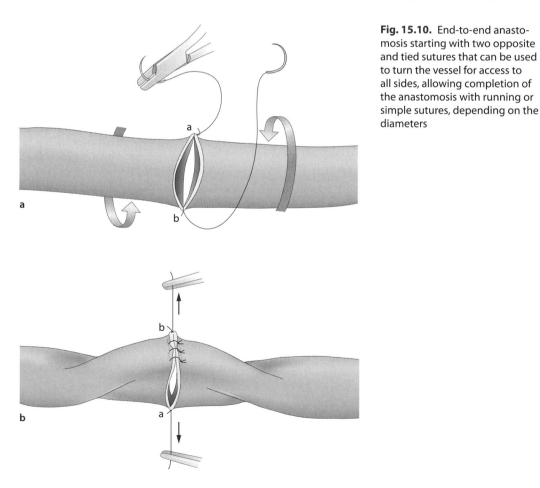

Fig. 15.10. End-to-end anastomosis starting with two opposite and tied sutures that can be used to turn the vessel for access to all sides, allowing completion of the anastomosis with running or simple sutures, depending on the diameters

earlier, the distal edge should always be sutured with the needle from inside the lumen to guarantee that the distal intima is fixed. When anastomosing thinner arteries an interrupted suture can be preferable because it will diminish the risk of narrowing by a too-hard pull in a running suture.

The length of the graft is adjusted after the first anastomosis has been completed. A graft that is too long increases the risk of kinking, while one that is too short means an unacceptable tension in the anastomosis. Appropriate length is achieved if the graft is straightened with a vascular forceps until it is stretched and then cut at the level of the end of the other artery.

When choosing vascular prosthesis for a patch or interposition graft, larger arteries like the aorta, common and external iliacs, and the common femoral artery can be closed or reconstructed with synthetic prosthesis material. In the common femoral artery, however, an autologous vein can also be used. In vascular procedures distal to the groin an autologous vein should always be used as the first choice. The rationale is that synthetic material always has an increased thrombogenicity, which in combination with the low flow in thinner arteries leads to a higher risk for thrombosis and occlusion. But for reconstructing larger arteries with a higher flow, synthetic grafts work well.

In cases with increased risk for infection (i.e., contaminated traumatic injuries or vascular reconstructions performed in association with intestinal injuries or disease), the choice of prosthetic material is more challenging. A synthetic prosthesis always implies risk of a complicating infection of the implanted synthetic material. Such an infection is very difficult to treat and usually requires the graft to be totally excised. A vein graft is more resistant to infection, but these also carry a risk for erosion and serious bleeding. The basic principle is to always avoid synthetic grafts when there is increased risk of infection and to use an autologous vein as the first chose. Exceptions are procedures on larger arteries such as the aorta and iliacs, and if synthetic prostheses are used in such a situation, prolonged antibiotic therapy should be considered.

15.8.1 Autologous Vein

The most commonly used vein is the greater saphenous vein. Other alternatives are the lesser saphenous, cephalic, and basilic veins. At all vein harvesting a maximally atraumatic technique should be used.

The vein is exposed by one or several longitudinal skin incisions and all branches are ligated. Be sure that the length harvested is long enough for the present purpose. Immediately after harvesting the vein graft should be flushed clean of all remaining blood with a heparin solution 10 units/ml, in which it can be preserved until it is used. Veins usually have a pronounced contractility, causing them to shrink considerably when they are handled during exposure and harvest. Before a vein is used as an arterial substitute it should be checked for leaks. By gently injecting heparin solution and simultaneously occluding the outflow, remaining open branches or other injuries causing leakage can be revealed and fixed with 4-0 ligatures and 6-0 or 7-0 vascular sutures, respectively. When ligating a branch it is important to avoid "tenting" of the vein because this might cause narrowing and stenosis. For the same reason, all other leaks should be sealed with sutures placed in the long axis of the vessel. Note that if the vein is to be reversed, the larger end of the vein should consequently be anastomosed distally to eliminate the flow-obstructing effect of the valves. The technique for preparing an autologous vein patch and an interposition graft is shown in Fig. 15.11.

15.8.2 Synthetic Vascular Prosthesis

Synthetic vascular prostheses are available mainly in two materials: polyester or ePTFE (expanded PTFE). Both materials are available as straight tube and bifurcation grafts in different diameters ranging from 6 to 12 mm for the tubes and from 14 to 26 mm for the bifurcated grafts, in which the limb has half the diameter. Both materials are also available as sheets from which suitable patches can be cut.

Polyester prostheses are most commonly used in the aortoiliac region and are available as knitted material (which is the most common) and woven. The knitted version is permeable to blood, whereas

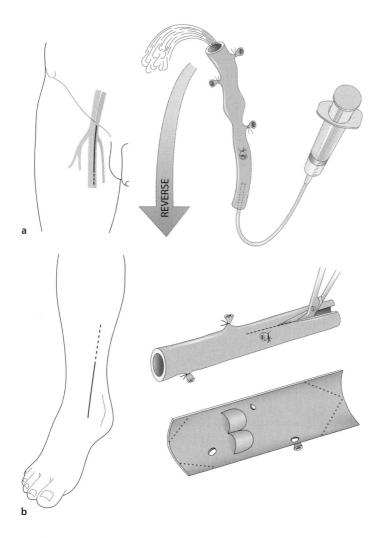

Fig. 15.11. Harvest of autologous vein for graft and patch. **a** Saphenous vein graft. A longitudinal incision over the vein starts in the groin and is elongated according to individual requirements. All branches are ligated and divided. The vein is harvested and flushed with heparinized glucose or saline. It must be reversed when used as an arterial substitute. **b** The greater saphenous vein at the ankle is usually sufficient and is exposed through an incision just anterior to the medial malleolus. All branches are ligated. The harvested vein is cut longitudinally and the ends trimmed. Be cautious and turn the patch so that the valves do not obstruct the flow

the latter is tight. Nowadays the knitted grafts are mostly available coated, which means they are impregnated with collagen or albumin in order to be sealed to blood. This type of coated knitted graft is the most commonly used.

If a noncoated knitted graft is chosen, it is extremely important to "preclot" it to avoid extensive leakage through the graft wall: Prior to heparinization, 20–30 ml of the patient's own blood is aspirated through an arterial puncture. The blood is immediately used to impregnate the vascular prosthesis. When the blood coagulates between the knits, the prosthesis will be sealed. If this step is forgotten, although the prosthesis will slowly seal after implantation, it will do so usually only after extensive bleeding.

PTFE is a porous but tight material very suitable for vascular prosthesis. It can also be used as an arterial substitute infrainguinally to perform an above-knee or even a below-knee femoropopliteal bypass. PTFE is possibly somewhat more resistant to infection than polyester is.

15.9 Veins

Surgical operations on veins require special and careful attention to technique because of the veins' thin wall structure and vulnerability. This is, naturally, particular important in emergent trauma cases. An iatrogenic or traumatic venous lesion can very easily be dramatically enlarged by just a slight pull with gauze in an attempt to control the bleeding. This vulnerability to injury is also why vascular clamps should be avoided for controlling veins. Instead, a piece of gauze of appropriate size on a straight clamp is carefully applied in a right angle over the vein on both sides of the lesion. A complete dissection with application of vessel-loops is rarely needed. The lesion can usually be directly repaired with a simple or running suture in the direction that causes the least degree of narrowing.

Smaller and midsize veins can be ligated. Reconstruction of injured veins is recommended for larger unpaired veins such as the vena cava and iliac and femoral veins; see Chapters 5 (p. 58) and 9 (p. 113). If suturing is insufficient and grafting is necessary due to a more extensive injury autologous material is the first choice, just as in repair of arterial injuries. If a graft with a larger diameter is needed, a spiral graft can be created from a longitudinally opened greater saphenous vein (see Fig. 15.12).

Technically challenging diffuse venous bleeding, such as in the pelvic region, can often be treated by a combination of applying a hemostatic agent (Table 15.2) and packing the bleeding with lots of dressings. The pressure in veins is low, and bleeding usually stops within 15–30 min. (The technique is further described on p. 152.) In a life-threatening situation, most veins, including the vena cava, can be ligated with reasonable consequences (e.g., swelling of limbs).

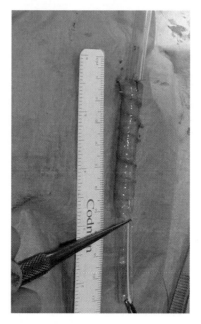

Fig. 15.12. Spiral graft technique to create a graft of larger diameter for replacing vein segments. A saphenous vein is cut longitudinally and sutured in a spiral fashion over plastic tubing used as a stent

NOTE

Veins are much more vulnerable than arteries. But the low venous pressure makes it possible to handle even severe venous bleeding and injuries with hemostatic agents and packing.

Table 15.2. Listing of local hemostatic agents and their characteristics

Agent	Application, examples	Special characteristics
Collagen	Oozing in anastomosis	
Oxygenated cellulose	Oozing in anastomosis	
Polyethylene glycol	Oozing in anastomosis	Works better on dry surfaces; polymerization in 60 s
Thrombin with or without gelatin	Larger bleeding in anastomosis	Expands about 20%; polymerization 3 min; ongoing bleeding necessary for access to fibrinogen
Fibrin glue	Diffuse bleeding	Frozen, must be thawed; spray covers larger areas

■ 15.10 Other

■ 15.10.1 Drains

Drains are rarely used after elective vascular procedures. However, they may be useful after emergency procedures in the neck and the legs to detect postoperative bleeding requiring intervention and to evacuate blood to minimize the risk of hematoma development with its increased risk for infection. Care should be taken to place the tube in a way that does not compress a vascular graft. The drain is recommended to be active. Removal of the drain shall be considered on the 1st postoperative day. Intraabdominal drains after emergency aortic surgery are rarely used.

■ 15.10.2 Infection Prophylaxis

Careful atraumatic technique and an optimal route of dissection, avoiding lymph glands and vessels, are important prophylactic measures for minimizing infection. Prophylactic antibiotics should be administered to patients with infected ulcerations or wounds and groin dissections and when synthetic prostheses are implanted. They are also generally recommended in all emergency procedures. Local protocols vary, but cloxacillin 2 g or cefuroxime 1.5 g are frequently used as a single preoperative dose given intravenously. The dose should be repeated every 3–4 h if open surgery is still going on.

Subject Index